THE
body clock
diet

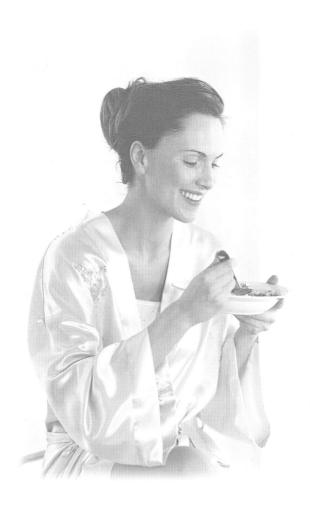

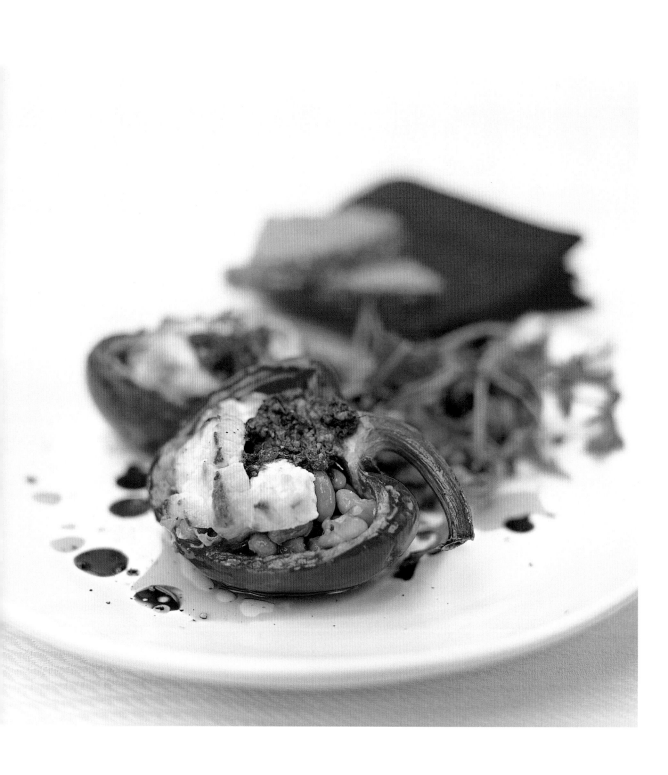

THE
body clock
diet

It's not only what you eat,
but when you eat it...

Lyndel Costain

hamlyn

First published in Great Britain in 2005 by
Hamlyn, a division of Octopus Publishing
Group Ltd
2–4 Heron Quays, London E14 4JP

Distributed in the United States and
Canada by Sterling Publishing Co., Inc.
387 Park Avenue South, New York,
NY 10016-8810

ISBN 0 600 61093 4

EAN 9780600610939

A CIP catalogue record for this book is
available from the British Library

Printed and bound in China

10 9 8 7 6 5 4 3 2 1

Disclaimer
While the author has made every effort
to provide accurate and up-to-date
information, the sciences of
chronobiology and weight control are
continuously evolving. This book contains
general guidance only and is not meant
to replace the advice you would get from
your doctor. You should always consult a
doctor, dietitian or other healthcare
professional for individualized health and
weight-control advice.

contents

introduction

Congratulations on deciding to get into shape and look after yourself! After all, it is not so easy these days, thanks to an abundance of tempting, high-calorie foods on offer, our more sedentary lifestyles, not to mention the time pressures and stress that constantly surround us. Combine all this with a body naturally designed to overeat when food is plentiful and to work best when it follows regular rhythms, and it is no wonder that our 'diets' fail, our exercise routines slip and our weight keeps going up.

Do you want to lose weight? If so, you are definitely not alone. At least three in five adults in western countries are now overweight or obese; in fact, a fifth are so overweight that it could shorten their lifespan by nine years. More and more children are overweight too – in the last 11 years obesity rates in children aged 5–16 in the UK have tripled.

Much of this is down to the effects of our modern 'weight-promoting' environment. Not only does it encourage us to be less active and to eat more, it also throws us out of sync with our body's natural cycles and regulators, making it much harder to manage our weight.

The body clock diet will help you take charge and regain control, right now and into the future.

How to use this book

The body clock diet provides a blueprint for healthy weight loss and ongoing healthy living. Packed with plenty of tips, advice and nutritional know-how, it also comes with a delicious 14-day menu plan (plus seven days of vegetarian menu plans) which you can use to get you started.

The menu plans, which provide three meals and two to three snacks daily, are nutritionally balanced and calorie-controlled to make things easy for you. You can mix and match breakfasts, lunches, evening meals and snacks from menu plans on different days, or swap lunch for your evening meal if that suits you better. Make sure you take note of the motivational and practical tips that accompany each menu plan too.

Before you start, complete the body clock questionnaires on pages 36–37 and read through the guidance given on pages 38–41 to ensure you get off to the very best start towards a slimmer, healthier you.

Each daily menu plan provides around 1,500 calories, a level at which most women will lose around 0.5 kg (1 lb) a week. You can lose more if you're also more active, but the healthy level is no more than 0.5–1 kg (1–2 lb) a week. Pages 54–55 have advice on how to put together your own meal plans or adjust your calorie intake to suit your individual needs. This can be especially helpful for men and very active women.

Now read more about how and why the body clock approach can work for you.

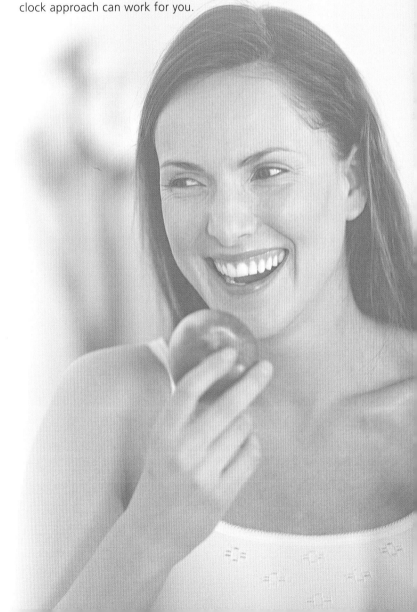

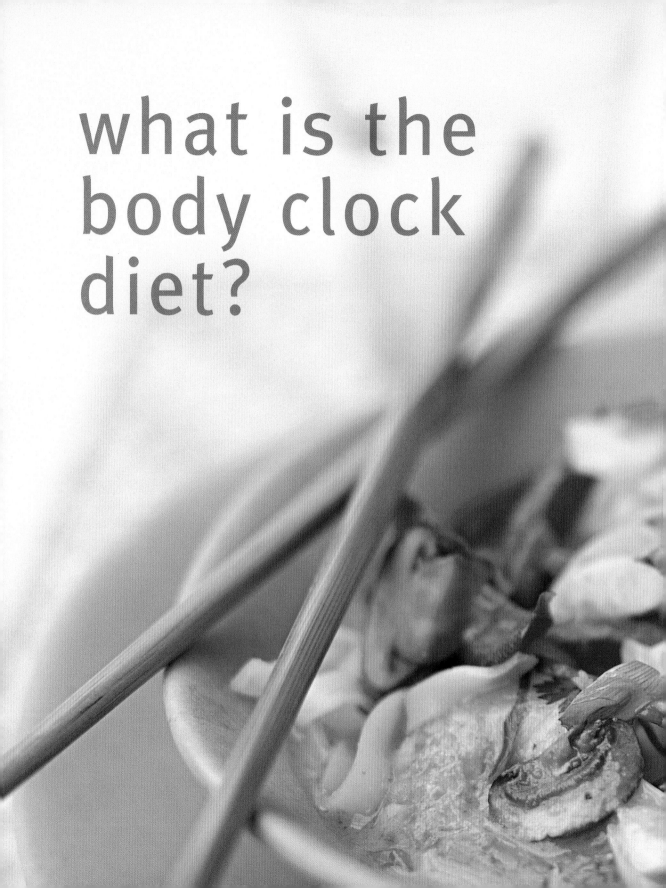

what is the body clock diet?

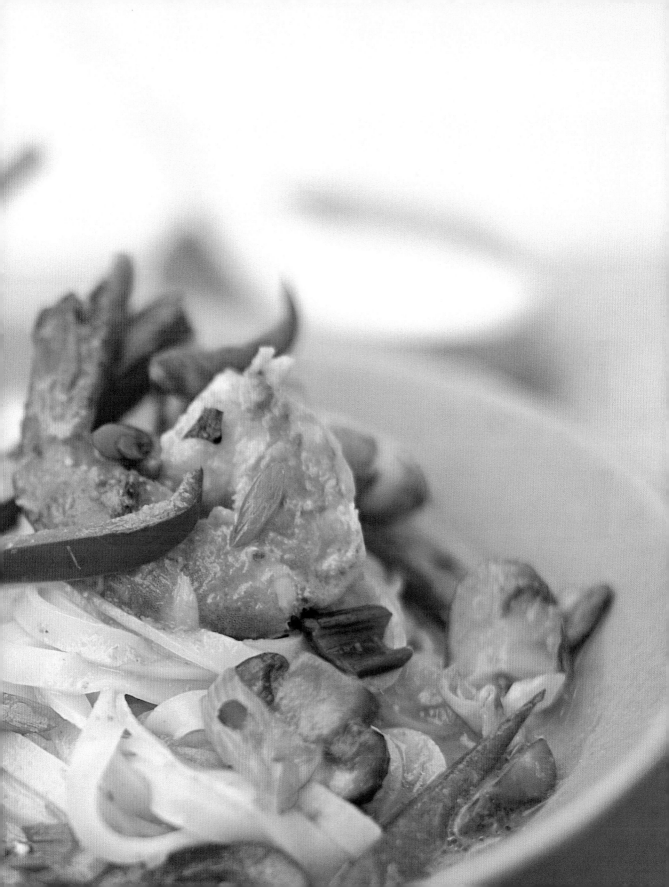

the body clock approach – an overview

The body clock diet aims to keep you in harmony with your body's natural rhythms. These 'circadian' (sir-kay-dee-in) rhythms (see page 12) are controlled by your in-built body clock and affect basic bodily functions such as your sleep/ wake-up cycle, your metabolism, your appetite, as well as your energy levels.

The trouble is that we can easily knock our body clocks out of sync. Erratic eating, shift work, strict diets, travel, stress or a few late nights can all take their toll. That is why it is important to find out about your body clock so that you can learn to live in harmony with it.

Living in tune with your body's natural rhythms, eating the right foods at the right time, is a key to good health – and that includes weight control.

The body clock diet and you
The body clock diet and its meal plans have been designed to help you not simply lose weight, but also improve your energy levels and sleep patterns, and manage your mood and food cravings. It will also help you get in touch with when and why you eat, allowing you to address the thoughts and actions that have sabotaged past efforts at losing weight.

This book introduces you to not just another 'diet', but a path to a new, healthy way of eating and living. There are no gimmicks, no unrealistic restrictions and no lists of forbidden foods, just a reliable approach to help you nourish body, mind and soul.

Following the advice given in this book will help you to lose up to 0.5–1 kg (1–2 lb) a week and find a weight that is right and realistic for you to 'settle' at. Although there is no magic wand to wave and no one has all the answers about weight loss, you will find here guidelines based on what research currently suggests is most effective for body rhythm and weight control. And because everyone is different, you can try out and tweak these guidelines to develop the strategies that suit you best.

TAKE IT EASY

A healthy weight loss is no more than 0.5–1 kg (1–2 lb) a week. You can achieve this easily by cutting down on a few calories and by being more active on a regular basis.

Health benefits

Losing a modest amount of weight reduces your risk of common health problems such as:

- Type 2 diabetes
- High blood pressure and stroke
- Heart disease
- High 'LDL' or 'bad' cholesterol
- Back or joint pain
- Osteoarthritis
- Certain cancers, e.g. breast, prostate
- Poor fertility and polycystic ovarian syndrome (cysts on the ovaries that can cause infertility)
- Sleep apnoea (when you stop breathing for very short periods during sleep)
- Low mood and self-esteem

Ten ticks of the body clock

Achieving lasting weight loss is about making long-term lifestyle changes. It is also about overcoming the barriers that have been stopping you from making these changes and reaching a healthier weight. The body clock approach will equip you with the knowledge and confidence to get these issues sorted, once and for all. So tick your way to success …

1 Believe in yourself

2 Be realistic, and value your achievements no matter how large or small

3 Stay aware of the 'weight-promoting' environment (see pages 6 and 17). Keeping a diary helps

4 Enjoy regular meals and planned snacks, starting with breakfast

5 Move more, more often, every day

6 Stop, think and really choose before you eat

7 When things go off track, forgive yourself and move on

8 Make a good night's sleep a priority

9 Reward your progress and have regular 'me-time' – starting now

10 Get ongoing support and encouragement from a friend, partner, health professional, club or from this book! (see page 40)

OBESE OR OVERWEIGHT?

A person is defined as overweight if their Body Mass Index (BMI) (see page 38) is between 25 and 29.9. Obesity is defined as a BMI of 30 or more.

your body clock and you

Have you ever wondered why you become tired at night and want to sleep? Or why you find it difficult to concentrate at work in the early afternoon? Or why food cravings strike at a certain time of day? The answers lie in the recently discovered and evolving science of chronobiology.

Chronobiology is the study of in-built circadian rhythms. It has been found that these rhythms affect hundreds of basic bodily functions, including your sleep/wake-up cycle, body temperature, blood pressure, metabolic rate, alertness, appetite, digestion, energy levels, sex drive and body repair. They do this by regulating hormones and other chemical messengers in the brain and in parts of the body. The word 'circadian' comes from the Latin – circa diem – meaning 'about a day'. This is because circadian rhythms have a cycle that lasts just over 24 hours, in harmony with the earth's 24-hour rotation.

Our circadian rhythms are part of our genetic make-up and are driven by an internal body clock so powerful that it cannot be reset simply whenever you want to. Studies have been made of human volunteers cut off from the outside world and exposed only to artificial light. After a few days their bodies still naturally followed cycles, including sleeping and eating. This helps to explain how our bodies keep functioning in a regular and restorative way, day to day, and as seasons change.

What drives the body clock?

The master body clock or 'chief controller' for circadian rhythms is a cluster of nerve cells called the suprachiasmatic nucleus (SCN). It is found in a part of the brain called the hypothalamus (see diagram opposite) and sends signals to other parts of the brain. It also coordinates a relay of messages from smaller body clocks located in different parts of the body, for example in the liver and skin.

One of the key roles of the SCN is to prepare your body for sleep by triggering the release of the chemical messenger melatonin from the pineal gland at the base of the brain. Melatonin works by slightly lowering your body temperature, making you feel drowsy. It also triggers the orchestration of other hormone levels, such as cortisol, growth hormone, leptin, insulin and anti-diuretic hormone, helping your body to rest, detoxify and restore itself. In the early morning hours, melatonin levels start to fall, gearing your body to wake up – thanks again to your body clock.

Are all body clocks in time?

While most people have sociable circadian rhythms, helping them to sleep at night and be alert during the day, some would say that they are either 'morning' or 'night' people – affectionately known as 'larks' or 'owls'. Larks prefer to get up early and greet the day; owls prefer to stay in bed later and are active late into the evening. Then again, some people do best with seven hours sleep, while others need nine. Despite these individual differences, as a rule people's body clocks generally follow similar rhythms.

Occasionally, however, someone's body clock becomes so out of sync that sleep and quality of life are affected (see page 14). Then there is travel across time zones and shift work, which also play havoc with your body clock (see page 15).

Your body clock in action

6–8 am   Body prepares for activity. Temperature rises, the stress hormone cortisol rises and peaks, as does neuropeptide Y (see page 21), triggering the need for a carbohydrate-rich breakfast. The immune system is at its weakest.

9–11am   Adrenaline and temperature rises. Glucose metabolism optimal. Peak of mental alertness.

12–1 pm   Appetite stimulated, ready for next meal.

1–3 pm   Lowest energy point, body temperature drops slightly – the post-lunch dip. Cravings likely.

3–4 pm   Body temperature and adrenaline levels rise. Cortisol peak

again. Good time for concentrating and working. Pain threshold is high.

4–6/7 pm   Coordination, stamina, body temperature, metabolism and adrenaline peak – the body's best time for exercise. Then it is ready to refuel. Mood is good.

8–11 pm   Body temperature and adrenaline fall and, preparing for sleep, body begins to produce melatonin. Mental and physical fatigue begin to show.

11–4 am   Need for food, drink and urine output minimized through the night. Body starts to restore and repair for the day ahead. Metabolism-regulating growth hormone rises and peaks when we enter 'deep sleep'. Melatonin stays high; blood pressure and heart rate low.

4–6 am   Body temperature and alertness are at their lowest, to promote good sleep and mental restoration.

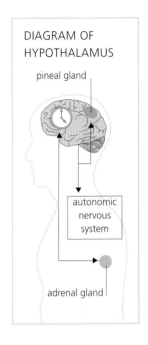

DIAGRAM OF HYPOTHALAMUS

pineal gland

autonomic nervous system

adrenal gland

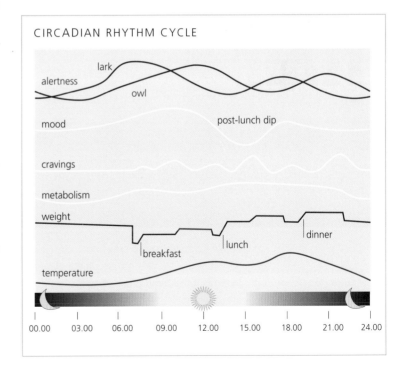

CIRCADIAN RHYTHM CYCLE

when body clocks run to different times

SEASONAL DEPRESSION

Body clock upsets are thought to contribute to seasonal affective disorder (SAD), a form of depression in which winter low-light levels lead to low mood, sleep problems, food cravings and lethargy.

Imagine what life was like 200 years ago in rural, pre-industrial times. You would have gone to bed not long after dark, risen and worked with the light and been guided by your circadian rhythms. In developed industrialized societies we live in an environment that is totally different from the one we evolved in – we use alarm clocks, fly across time zones, work through the night or stay up watching television or partying!

All this is at odds with your body clock's in-built drive to harmonize and optimize mental and physical functions during the day and the body-restoring night, which can mean upsets in sleep patterns, energy levels, appetite – and weight control.

According to recent research in the UK and USA, genetic differences mean that some people naturally have circadian cycles that run one to two hours ahead or behind most people, but are still quite healthy, and follow a regular rhythm. These are the 'larks', who just love waking early but cannot stay up late, and the 'owls', who lie in for as long as they can, then come into their own in the evening.

If you are a lark or an owl, you can try to tailor your work and lifestyle to your personal highs and lows of alertness. Or you can try to advance or push back your body clock with the tips opposite. These tips are also useful if your body clock has been reset by a few unusually early mornings or late nights, say after a weekend when you go to bed and get up much later than usual.

Body clock disorders

In rare cases, the body clock can be upset by an inherited disorder known as delayed or advanced sleep phase syndrome. People with this condition may sleep best from 4 am until noon if it is 'delayed', or from 7 pm to 3 am if 'advanced', despite their best efforts to sleep at regular times. If you think this is a problem for you, do talk to your doctor.

How to adjust your body clock

If you are a lark and need to stay up later, for a few days:

■ Spend time outside in the afternoon or early evening

■ Increase evening activity

■ Sleep with blinds or curtains closed

■ Lie and rest in bed until it is time to get up if you wake early

■ Delay meal times in line with later bed- and get-up times

If you are an owl (or have had a few late nights out) and need to get up earlier:

■ Avoid any stimulating activities in the evenings – try and relax before bed

■ Try sleeping with blinds or curtains open

■ Walk outside shortly after waking up

■ Get up at the same time every day – set an alarm clock

■ Adjust meal times in line with earlier bed- and get-up times

Jet lag and shift work

When you fly across a few time zones, you disrupt your circadian rhythms and end up with that uncomfortable feeling known as 'jet lag'. For example, if you fly from London to New York, you 'lose' six hours. Of course you will feel tired when the alarm rings at 8 am the next morning because, according to your body's clock, it is still 2 am.

It usually takes several days for your body's cycles to adjust to the new time. But you can help it along by using strategies similar to those for the 'larks'

and 'owls', depending on whether you have travelled back or forwards across time zones (see page 72).

If you do shift work, you are often working against powerful sleep-regulating cues such as sunlight. This means you can feel drowsy during shifts, and sleep problems are common. Some people may suffer digestive upsets and mood, weight, blood sugar and even heart health problems. You are also out of tune with your body's optimal performance times, which increases the risk of errors or accidents.

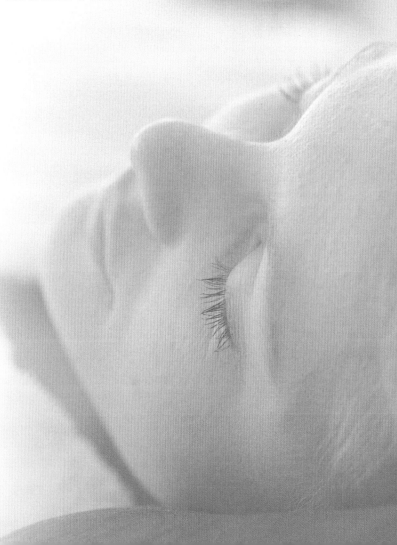

SHIFT WORK SOLUTIONS

Shift-related fatigue can be helped by having bright lights in the workplace, minimizing shift changes, taking planned naps and exercise breaks and having a regular, healthy meal pattern (see page 20).

food –
your life-sustaining fuel

Food is your fuel. It provides the energy you need for metabolism and every bodily activity – breathing, digestion, mental activity, muscle function, heart beats, hormone production, temperature regulation, immunity, movement and exercise. You must eat, quite literally, to stay alive. The quality of your fuel mix is also essential for a healthy body and mind. The body clock way of eating, with its delicious meal plans, will provide that mix for you.

Food is made up of carbohydrates, fats, protein, fibre, vitamins, minerals and water. Energy in food is measured in calories and is provided by fats, carbohydrates (from both sugars and starches), protein and alcohol. Fat contains twice the calories of carbohydrate or protein and makes food taste very more-ish, which is why eating a lot of high-fat foods makes it easy to gain weight.

Vitamins and minerals are needed in relatively tiny amounts, but are still essential for growth and development, and to regulate the body's chemical processes and functions. Some minerals also have a structural role, for example calcium in bones and teeth.

Fuel your life

Healthy weight loss involves getting the nutrients you need, feeling positive about helping your health and optimizing your metabolism and body composition (lose fat and tone muscle). It also must be do-able in day-to-day life.

This means not just following yet another diet, but developing new skills and attitudes to keep the weight off. In the body clock approach, rather than simply aiming for a certain weight, you work to identify why you have been finding it hard to get to or maintain a healthier weight. Once you have mastered this, coupled with the real belief that you can manage your weight, you will find that maintaining your ideal weight becomes less of a chore and just a natural part of your lifestyle.

The facts about losing weight

Your weight is regulated by the difference between the calories you consume and the calories burned by your metabolism and physical activity.

PLANT-DERIVED EXTRAS

Foods derived from plants contain a wide range of beneficial compounds called 'phytochemicals'. Many of these work as antioxidants, protecting the body from the harmful effects of unstable free radicals (see page 19).

When these two are in balance, your weight remains stable. When you consume more calories than you burn, you will store them and gain weight; and when you consume less than you burn, you will burn fat and lose weight.

Your internal 'drive to eat' or hunger is largely controlled by a part of the brain called the hypothalamus, which is where your body clock sits too (see pages 13 and 21). Of course, if eating was tightly regulated, then few people would be overweight! But we all have different genes, and these internal 'controllers' are easily overridden. For example, in the developed world we live in a food-filled environment, and you may find you want to eat for all sorts of different reasons, such as boredom or for comfort. You may also have an uneasy relationship with food, for example comfort or binge eating, that needs a bit of sorting out.

Slow but sure

Body weight typically fluctuates on a day-to-day basis. You know that shock/horror feeling when you weigh yourself in the evening, perhaps after a meal out, and it looks as though you have gained several pounds since you weighed yourself that morning? Don't panic – this is due to fluid changes not fat changes.

Don't be fooled either by very rapid weight loss in the first week or so of a crash or low-carbohydrate diet. When calorie intake is initially cut right back, the body's carbohydrate stores in the liver and muscles (known as glycogen) are used up. Glycogen is stored with three times its weight in water, meaning

that rapid losses of 2–3 kg (4½–6½ lb) in a few days are possible. But these weight losses will be short-lived as stores are quickly refilled as soon as you go back to your usual eating habits.

True weight change happens over a longer period of time than a week or two. Most light to moderately active men will lose weight (at around 0.5 kg/1 lb a week) on 1,800–2,000 calories a day and most women will lose weight on 1,500 calories a day. Those with a more active lifestyle (or if they are very overweight) will lose up to 1 kg (2 lb) a week.

CALORIE COUNT

To lose weight, you need to consume fewer calories than you burn in a sustained way. For example, 0.5 kg (1 lb) of body fat contains 3,500 calories, so to lose this in a week, you need a daily 500 calorie deficit (7 x 500 = 3,500).

nourish your body and mind

The body clock diet is based on cutting-edge healthy eating guidelines with an optimal mix of protein, nutritious carbohydrates and healthy fats, embedded with vital vitamins, minerals and antioxidants. Here are the basics.

Healthy eating basics

Healthy eating is about enjoying more of the foods that suit your individual needs and that protect and nourish your body. With time they will become your natural choice. Each day, choose a healthy proportion from each of the different food groups (see pages 54–55). These are:

■ At least five portions of **fruit and vegetables**. Fresh, frozen, canned, dried and juiced all count (except potatoes) – they are full of vitamins, minerals and protective antioxidants. (Note – only count juice once towards your five a day.)

■ Healthy **energy** foods such as bread, pasta, rice, potatoes, cereals and noodles. Make them part of meals and choose satisfying wholegrain types for extra vitamins, minerals and fibre.

■ Two to three servings of reduced-fat **milk and dairy products** (or calcium-fortified soya alternatives) for protein, calcium and B vitamins.

■ Two to three moderate servings of **protein**-rich foods, such as lean meat, fish, chicken, eggs, pulses, tofu, nuts or seeds. These also provide iron, B vitamins, zinc, magnesium and selenium.

■ Modest amounts of **unsaturated oils and spreads** for vitamins D and E and essential fats. Keep to small amounts of fatty or sugary foods. Limit salt too as a high intake can raise blood pressure.

More about nutrition

Protein

Protein is vital for growth, repair of body tissues and to build hormones and other chemical messengers that regulate body processes. It can also provide energy (calories) for fuel. Protein is very useful for regulating your appetite too. In fact, studies suggest that it is more satisfying than carbohydrate or fat, helping you feel fuller for longer.

Carbohydrate and fibre

There are three main types of carbohydrate in food: sugars, starches and fibre. Glucose is a type of sugar that circulates in the blood and is the easiest carbohydrate for your body to turn into energy. Starchy carbohydrate is found in foods like pasta, potatoes, bread, rice, cereals and pulses. These are important, especially wholegrain varieties, as they contain a range of vital nutrients. So forget low-carbohydrate diets – letting healthy carbs into your life makes weight control easier and promotes long-term health.

Fibre comes in two main forms. 'Insoluble' fibre is found mainly in bran-based cereals, wholemeal bread and most vegetables. It works like a sponge and soaks up water in the bowel. Not getting enough can lead to constipation. 'Soluble fibre' is found in pulses, oats, barley, rye and most fruit. Its gummy characteristics help to regulate the levels of cholesterol and glucose in your blood. Foods rich in soluble fibre tend to have a low glycaemic index (see page 22), which means they break down into glucose slowly. Fibre can also keep the bacteria in your bowel in harmonious balance.

Fat

You need some fat in your diet to absorb fat-soluble vitamins A, D, E and K, build cell membranes and provide 'essential' fats that the body cannot make. You also need some fat stores to insulate and cushion the body, and make vital hormones. Yes, women need curves! The trick is to get a good balance of the right fats, as different fats affect our health in different ways.

Eating too much food rich in saturated or trans fats, such as fatty meats, cakes, biscuits and full-fat dairy foods, can raise blood cholesterol levels, while switching to beneficial unsaturated fats found in olive and rapeseed oil, nuts and avocados can lower them. Omega-3 fats, found mainly in oily fish, help to keep the heart

and nervous and immune systems healthy, and can even influence mood.

Phytochemicals

Found in fruit, vegetables, wholegrains, nuts and seeds, phytochemicals ('plant chemicals') are not true nutrients, but do have properties that keep the immune system strong and reduce the risk of long-term problems like heart disease, cancers and lung disorders. Many function as antioxidants by mopping up excess 'free radicals', which are unstable molecules that whiz around the body with the potential to damage healthy cells.

WHAT'S A PORTION?

For information on portions and serving sizes, see page 54.

THE BALANCE OF GOOD HEALTH

The diagram below shows the five main food groups in healthy proportions.

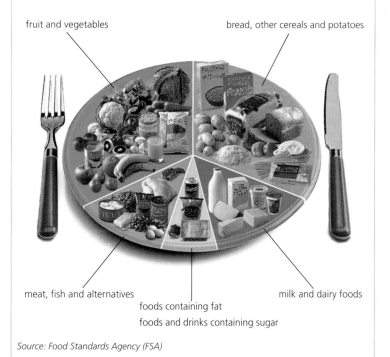

fruit and vegetables

bread, other cereals and potatoes

meat, fish and alternatives

foods containing fat
foods and drinks containing sugar

milk and dairy foods

Source: Food Standards Agency (FSA)

eating regularly

Now that you know more about circadian rhythms, it should come as no surprise that the timing of your meals is a vital part of the body clock approach to weight control. Studies suggest that regular meal times could even help reset an out-of-sync body clock.

The more you can stay in tune with your body's rhythms, the better it is for your digestion, hormone balance, appetite, energy levels and mood.

Why regular meals?

If you often follow strict diets, skip meals due to lack of time or eat for comfort when you're not really hungry, you override the actions of chemical messengers that signal and regulate your natural feelings of hunger and fullness. This makes it difficult for your body to recognize how much food it needs, and when. The end result can be bingeing, high-fat snacking or eating all evening after a day without food! Eating meals and snacks at a similar time each day enables you to get back in tune with your body's appetite and energy cycles. Regular meals help you to:
■ Keep your blood insulin and sugar levels on an even keel
■ Think less about food between meals
■ Be less interested in high-fat snacks between meals
■ Let your body learn when it is time for your next meal
■ Feel comfortably hungry when it comes to meal times
■ Find it easier to recognize when you have had enough to eat at a meal, and stop eating

What is regular eating?

Regular eating is not leaving more than three or four hours between meals or snacks. So set times for when you will eat, for example around 8 am for breakfast, 10.30 am for a snack, 1 pm for lunch, 4 pm snack, 7.30 pm for an evening meal. If you are a 'lark', your meals might start and end earlier; if you are an 'owl', they will probably start later.

Initially, having regular meals can feel strange or impractical, but try your best and you will soon adapt. Once your regular eating puts you back in tune with your body clock, you will feel more in control of what and how much you eat.

What to eat, when

Your appetite is regulated by a part of the brain called the hypothalamus. It links in with your body clock and takes account of information from nerves, hormones and messengers from other parts of the brain. It also links to the digestive system to find out how much you have eaten recently, your blood sugar levels and how much fuel you have stored.

Breakfast

To function at its best, your body likes a regular supply of energy and nutrients, starting with breakfast. Overnight, and under the control of your body clock, your body has been silently repairing and restoring by tapping into your fuel stores, especially carbohydrates in the liver and muscle. To ensure that your stores are recharged for the day ahead, a messenger called neuropeptide Y (NPY) is released to trigger your desire for carbohydrates. Meanwhile, insulin, the hormone that invites blood sugar into cells for storage or to burn as fuel, is at its most efficient.

Studies from the Institute of Food Research in the UK have found that a high-carbohydrate breakfast optimizes morning mood and concentration. It also switches off NPY to stop carbohydrate cravings (see right). So breakfast really is a 'must have'!

A booster snack mid-morning will help balance blood insulin and sugar levels during your optimal concentration period. Choosing foods with a low glycaemic index (see page 23) ensures slow-release energy.

Lunchtime

This calls for satisfying 'alertness food' to get you through the post-lunch dip and stave off the effects of galanin, a chemical messenger that stimulates fat cravings. Galanin levels begin to rise after lunch and peak early evening, but making sure you have a good serving of protein combined with some healthy fats and carbohydrates at lunchtime will help to keep your cravings in check.

Mid- to late-afternoon, another 'slow-release' snack will keep your appetite regulators and you in control.

Dinner

The evening meal calls for a calming balance of nutrients to appease your hormones and gently refuel your body for its restorative functions overnight.

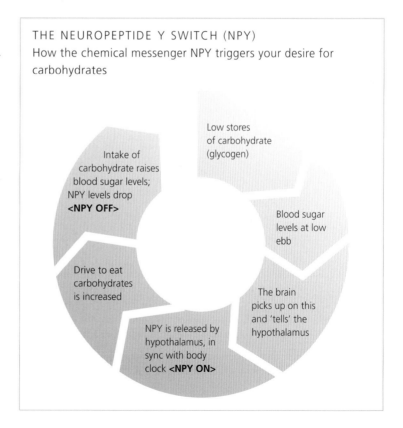

THE NEUROPEPTIDE Y SWITCH (NPY)
How the chemical messenger NPY triggers your desire for carbohydrates

Low stores of carbohydrate (glycogen)

Intake of carbohydrate raises blood sugar levels; NPY levels drop **<NPY OFF>**

Blood sugar levels at low ebb

Drive to eat carbohydrates is increased

The brain picks up on this and 'tells' the hypothalamus

NPY is released by hypothalamus, in sync with body clock **<NPY ON>**

let good carbs into your life – the glycaemic index

FIVE TOP TIPS FOR LOW-GI EATING

1 Include one low-GI food at each meal

2 Choose breakfast cereals based on oats or bran

3 Eat plenty of vegetables, fruit and pulses – at least five portions a day

4 Opt for wholegrain breads, preferably with visible seeds or grains

5 Use lower-GI varieties of potatoes and rice, such as basmati and wild rice

With constant hype around low-carbohydrate diets, it is easy to believe that pasta and potatoes are truly out of favour. But the real story is that not all carbohydrates are created equal.

Carbohydrates are digested to provide blood glucose (sugar) for fuel – potatoes, oats, wholegrain breads and cereals, pasta and noodles, for example, are all excellent sources of energy. On the other hand, carbohydrate-rich refined and sugary foods, like croissants, biscuits, fizzy drinks, pastries and sweets, are not such good choices.

From food to blood glucose

When we eat any carbohydrate-rich food, blood glucose levels rise and the hormone insulin is released, which encourages the body to store fat and shunts glucose into our cells where it is used to provide energy. The rate at which this happens depends on the food's glycaemic index (GI). This is a ranking of foods from 1 to 100 according to how quickly they break down to glucose in the bloodstream.

Foods that break down quickly in the body, for example, white rice, sweets and sugary cereals, have the highest GIs. High-GI foods raise blood glucose and insulin levels faster and higher, risking rebound crashes in blood sugar and cravings for the next food fix. In contrast, foods with a low GI break down slowly, releasing glucose and insulin calmly into the bloodstream.

GI: weight loss and health

So how can this help you to control your weight? There is increasing scientific evidence that low-GI foods help you feel fuller for longer and optimize levels of insulin in the blood. Research also suggests that low-GI and fibre-rich foods help to reduce hunger by affecting the release of appetite-regulating chemical messengers, such as GIP, GLP-1 and CCK, from the digestive system.

Healthier blood glucose and fat levels are two more key benefits of eating low-GI foods. Studies also link them to reduced risk of heart disease and type 2 diabetes, and better morning memory. The fibre content of most low-GI foods helps to keep the bowel regular, and promote a healthy balance of its bacteria, which in turn keeps you healthier. Low-GI foods also fuel exercise and make it easier to work out for longer (see page 58).

This is quite different from low-carbohydrate diet rules that restrict the very foods that nutrition research says protect your health and your weight. Yes, you should cut back on sugary and refined carbohydrates with a high GI and replace them with lower-GI alternatives for your nutritional health's sake, as well as your body clock's. But there is no need to go to low-carb extremes, and any rigid diet is just too difficult to sustain long term. Not to mention that a little of what you fancy really does do you some good (see page 26).

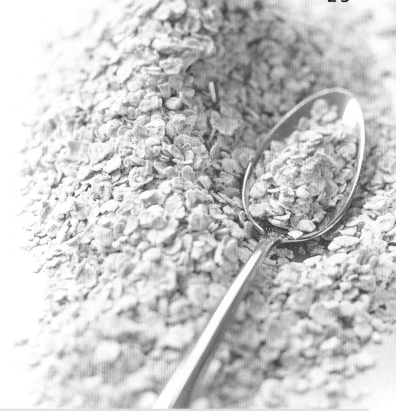

THE GLYCAEMIC INDEX OF COMMON FOODS

Low-GI foods have a GI less than 55, moderate GI is 55–69 and high GI is 70 or more.

High GI

Food	GI
Glucose	100
White rice, cooked	87
Baked potato	85
Cornflakes	84
Rice Krispies	82
Rice cakes	82
Jelly beans	80
Doughnut	76
French fries	75
White bread	70

Source: Adapted from Foster-Powell k et al, 'International tables of glycemic index and glycemic load values', American Journal of Clinical Nutrition 2002; 76 (1): 5–56.

Moderate GI

Food	GI
Wholemeal bread	69
Shredded Wheat	67
Pineapple	66
Sucrose (table sugar)	65
Rye bread	65
New potatoes, boiled	62
Ice cream	61
Digestive biscuits	59
Honey	58
Basmati rice	58
Pitta bread	57
Apricots	57
Sultanas	56
Bananas	55

Low GI

Food	GI
Sweet potatoes	54
Kidney beans, canned	52
Milk chocolate	49
Baked beans	48
Cracked wheat, cooked	48
Orange juice	46
Orange	44
Porridge	42
AllBran	42
Spaghetti, white, cooked	41
Apple	38
Yogurt, low-fat, fruit	33
Lentils, cooked	30
Peanuts	14

mood boosters

SWEET TEMPTATION

Chocolate may be the most popular food to improve mood – until the guilt sets in, making your good mood slump down into the doldrums. This shows just how powerful emotional responses to food can be. The body clock approach will help you to cope with those responses (see page 81).

You should well and truly have the message by now that your body clock plays a key role in regulating your health, weight and well-being. A lot of this is down to the way it orchestrates the ebb and flow of hormones and chemical messengers – things that also influence your mood. What, when and why you eat also has a huge impact on mood.

Feed your mind

The brain is made up of a complex network of nerve cells and is constantly active. Each cell needs oxygen and a cocktail of nutrients to function normally and build the neurotransmitters (chemical messengers) that allow nerve cells to communicate. A balanced and varied diet supplies the required raw ingredients, and the body clock way of eating makes sure you get them at the right time.

A lack of B vitamins has been linked to low mood in a range of studies, probably because they are needed to build the chemical messengers involved in thinking, alertness and feeling good, such as serotonin, adrenaline, dopamine and acetylcholine. Magnesium and vitamin C help build dopamine too. A lack of iron in the diet can lead to energy- and mood-sapping anaemia, a problem that affects around 1 in 10 women. The mineral selenium is needed to prevent anxiety, depression and tiredness. And omega-3 fats, found mainly in oily fish, seem to buffer the brain against depression, again through their effects on mood-regulating chemical messengers.

Carbs, sugar and serotonin

No doubt you have dived for the sweet stuff when the blues have hit or when your period is due if you are female (see page 80). After all, 97 per cent of women (and 68 per cent of men) report having food cravings, usually for sweet or fatty snacks such as chocolate, ice cream, crisps and pizza.

Yet a survey from the UK mental health charity MIND found that sweets, biscuits, fried food and coffee had the most negative impact on mood, while pasta, oily fish and fresh fruit were related to feelings of well-being. And when you look at the lists of foods rich in mood-boosting nutrients (see opposite), you will see that these findings make perfect sense.

Cravings for sweets and other carbohydrates have often been blamed on low levels of serotonin, a chemical messenger that helps to regulate mood (antidepressant medications often work by raising serotonin levels), as well as appetite and sleep. Serotonin is strongly tied in to your body clock, not least because melatonin, the light-sensitive sleep-inducing hormone (see page 12), is made from it. However, psychology experts now believe that while carbohydrate intake plays some role in regulating serotonin, the cravings we experience are dictated more by our emotional need for the food, and the comfort we know it brings (see page 81).

All this means that by recognizing food cravings you can learn to deal with them, and with time retrain the way your body and mind respond.

Food for happiness

The following nutrients help to maintain your feelings of well-being:
- Iron – from lean red meat, fortified cereals, oily fish and seafood, pulses
- Selenium – from fish and seafood, Brazil nuts, wholegrains
- B vitamins – from lean meat, fish, dairy foods, nuts, green leafy vegetables
- Magnesium – from fish, nuts, seeds, wholegrains, pulses
- Omega-3s – from oily fish (mackerel, trout, salmon, sardines, pilchards, swordfish, fresh tuna), omega-3-enriched eggs, rapeseed oil, linseeds, walnuts, tofu, pumpkin seeds

BEAT CRAVINGS WITH CARBS

The type of carbohydrate you eat can make coping with cravings that much easier. Sugary foods and drinks with a high GI (see page 23) give a quick blood sugar and mood boost, but you will soon be looking for the next one. Opt for low-GI foods and the sustained blood sugar and insulin rise will keep your appetite-regulating hormones in harmony.

LOW-GI BENEFITS

New research from the University of Swansea in Wales suggests that low-GI eating favours memory and mood. Low-GI foods also help to fuel exercise, which is one of the best mood boosters of all (see page 29).

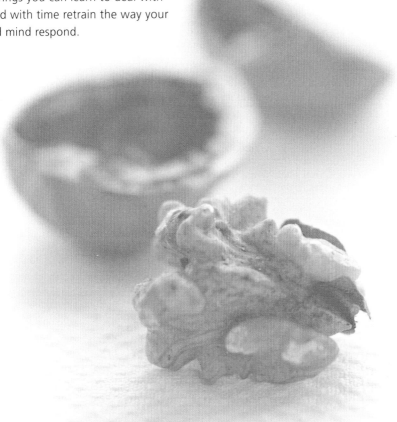

keeping it balanced

The body clock approach helps you to work with your body's natural rhythms both to feel great and to achieve the weight you want. A key part of that process is linked with how you think, feel and react.

To change your weight, you must also change your mind. You will become someone who feels good about themselves (starting now!) and truly believes in their ability to control their health and their weight. You will have the knowledge and confidence to do it and keep on believing that the changes you are making are worth keeping up – not just because they will keep you slimmer, but because you will feel fabulous.

A little of what you fancy
One of the many great things about the body clock diet is the lack of long lists of forbidden foods. All foods can fit (in moderation), but when you eat them can make a difference.

For example, that tempting chocolate bar is not wise during the daily post-lunch dip because it is a vulnerable time for energy lows and food cravings. But planning it into your diet when PMS

strikes (see page 81) may be just what you need. The satisfaction it provides can stop you craving, and eating, sugar all day long!

Eating healthily most of the time yet still making room for some of your really favourite foods is the key to long-term weight control and a happy, healthy relationship with food. Because of the modern environment we live in, where food is so abundant, just about everyone has to stop, think and make conscious choices about what they eat. And there is the key. Make a real choice about what you want to eat, then savour and enjoy it consciously and you won't feel deprived if it is less than you are used to.

When nothing is forbidden, you can either have a little, or none, now and some another day. This is what successful slimmers do. It also helps you to stay out of the destructive diet–binge cycle.

The diet–binge cycle
If you are forever trying the latest diet, avoid all sweet foods, obsessively count calories, then end up eating excessively, you may well be stuck in the diet–binge cycle. It does nothing for your self-esteem nor your belief that you can control your weight – or that you are

worth doing it for. Can you see yourself in there? If so, the body clock approach can help you break free.

Alcohol

Most of us like to enjoy a drink now and again, but keep in mind 'sensible' limits (see page 88). Lowering your alcohol consumption is not only good for your health and your weight, it also helps keep your body clock in sync. For example, a hangover has been likened to the body clock disruptions that bad jet lag brings (see pages 15 and 72) – and then there's the headache!

Remember that while drinking can help you get to sleep, it can also make you wake early. This is probably because alcohol disrupts the circadian rhythm of body temperature, as well as sleep-regulating chemical messengers such as serotonin.

What about caffeine?

It is vital to drink enough fluid during the day for both good health and weight control (see page 55), but you should take care with caffeine-containing drinks. Caffeine, found largely in coffee, tea, chocolate and cola, is a stimulant, so makes you feel alert. In fact, it can override the body clock's natural dips, helping you through the post-lunch dip or keeping you more alert during night shifts (see pages 15 and 62). The important thing is not to overdo it.

Some people are very sensitive to caffeine and know they need to avoid it. Others cope well, and even find it beneficial when enjoyed in moderation, for example, no more than three daily cups of brewed coffee or six cups of tea.

EFFECTS OF ALCOHOL

Alcohol has also been shown to decrease levels of leptin, a hormone that works to switch off hunger. This upset in leptin's normal circadian rhythms may add to post-drinking munchies, which are triggered by alcohol's ability to lower blood sugar levels.

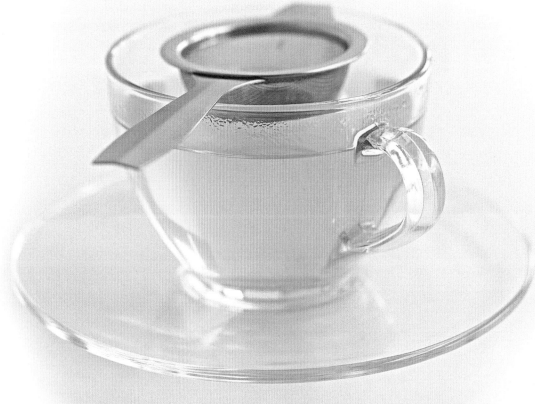

move more, more often

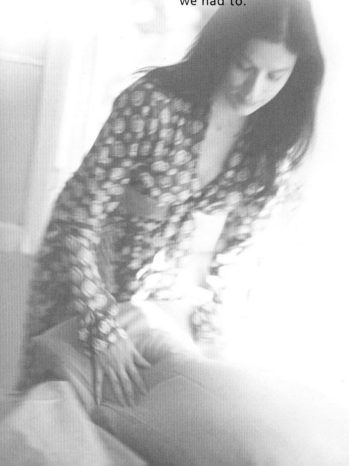

Gone are the days of saying 'I must do some exercise'! One of your new body clock mantras will be 'move more, more often'. Our bodies were designed to move regularly over the day, and as a result stay fit, strong and flexible enough to move swiftly when we had to.

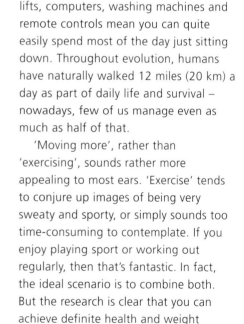

One of the key reasons behind the western world's obesity epidemic is the fact that we no longer need to move much in our day-to-day lives. Great as they are, labour-saving devices like cars, lifts, computers, washing machines and remote controls mean you can quite easily spend most of the day just sitting down. Throughout evolution, humans have naturally walked 12 miles (20 km) a day as part of daily life and survival – nowadays, few of us manage even as much as half of that.

'Moving more', rather than 'exercising', sounds rather more appealing to most ears. 'Exercise' tends to conjure up images of being very sweaty and sporty, or simply sounds too time-consuming to contemplate. If you enjoy playing sport or working out regularly, then that's fantastic. In fact, the ideal scenario is to combine both. But the research is clear that you can achieve definite health and weight benefits by fitting more movement into your day, for example, walking, using the stairs or even regular sex (see page 32).

Why bother?

When it comes to losing weight – and keeping it off – moving more is as important as fine-tuning what you eat and how you think. In fact, it is perhaps the most important predictor of long-term slimming success. Those who keep moving do best.

Being active boosts levels of your alertness hormones, adrenaline and noradrenaline (see page 30), and mood-regulating serotonin, and reduces the stress hormone cortisol. In short, losing weight with regular activity and a healthy diet improves 'out-of-whack' levels of hormones, blood sugar and appetite regulators, and promotes regular sleep – all changes that help to keep your body clock in harmony and your body trim.

Not only that, it helps you to feel good about yourself. And that in itself is vital to losing weight and staying in shape. If you do not like yourself before you have even started losing weight, then it is easy to feel that you are just not worth the effort involved in taking care of yourself. The end result is that any weight loss attempt is short-lived. Sound familiar?

Now, read this list and you will never doubt the benefits of moving more, more often again, because it helps you to:

■ Lose weight
■ Regulate your appetite
■ Improve your hormone balance
■ Release 'feel-good' endorphins
■ Beat food cravings and binges, including those linked to your monthly cycle
■ Preserve muscle strength (and metabolism) when weight is lost
■ Break through a weight plateau

■ Maintain your new healthy weight
■ Counteract the negative effects of shift work and jet lag
■ Boost your immunity and stave off coughs and colds
■ Reduce high blood pressure and lower risk of heart disease and stroke
■ Lower blood triglycerides and raise 'good' cholesterol
■ Reduce the risk of certain cancers
■ Reduce the risk of osteoporosis (brittle bones)
■ Improve insulin 'resistance' and reduce the risk of type 2 diabetes
■ Raise your self-esteem and confidence
■ Increase production of fat-burning, metabolism-managing growth hormone
■ Improve your mood and counteract depression
■ Sleep better
■ Manage stress and anxiety
■ Increase stamina and flexibility
■ Prevent lower back pain

Use a pedometer

Pedometers, available from sports shops or the Internet, are a fun way to motivate yourself to move more over the day. Clip it on to your belt or waistband and it counts how many steps you take each day.

Your first aim is to build up to 10,000 steps daily (that's equivalent to 30 minutes of moderate activity – see page 32). If you can then build up to 15,000 steps, or more, that's even better for fat burning. But the main thing is to move more than you were doing.

THE 'STRESS HORMONE' CORTISOL

Too much cortisol stimulates appetite, thickens your waist and dampens the immune system. Moving more keeps levels of cortisol under control.

daily routines – sleep and your body clock

MORNING MOVERS

If you like a regular work-out and morning is more convenient than late afternoon, then by all means stay with it – your body can adapt to perform best at the time you usually exercise. Just be sure to warm up properly to ensure your body is ready for action.

As you now know, your bodily functions follow a night and day rhythm. During the evening your body clock triggers a rise in melatonin, which lowers body temperature and adrenaline, making you feel tired and able to sleep. As morning approaches, your body clock triggers changes in the hormones adrenaline and noradrenaline, preparing your body and brain for the day ahead. These hormones make you alert and ready for action.

Being in tune with these cycles will help you to get maximum benefit from your eating and activity routines.

If you like to exercise regularly, you probably have a time and routine that works best for you. In that case, it's fine to stick with whatever you feel happy with. On the other hand, if you exercise at different times and often feel worn out, changing your routine so that you exercise in tune with your body clock may help. It can help you sleep better too, which is also vital for weight control (see opposite).

The best time to be active

When you first get up, your body temperature is still low – the changes to your metabolism that have helped you to sleep through the night are still having an effect. It is only later in the day that your temperature rises and peaks.

Studies have consistently shown that if you exercise late in the afternoon you will perform better than in the morning. This is because muscles are warm and more flexible, you react more quickly and your strength is at its peak. But these benefits are really only noticeable for fairly high-intensity exercise, like a full-on work-out or aerobic class.

Gentle 'moving more' exercise like walking, cycling or housework is fine whenever you want to do it. In fact, in the morning it helps you to wake up, feel alert and warm your body. The important thing is to just move more – so do it when it is best for you.

Exercise and sleep

Regular physical activity helps to keep your life in sync with your body clock, and with that comes a good night's sleep. But take care when you do it.

Since exercise releases stimulating adrenaline, exercising late at night or within a few hours of bedtime could stop you nodding off.

Your body performs best late in the afternoon, but if you do exercise at that time of the day and are having trouble sleeping, then recent research suggests exercising earlier in the day can help you ease into sleep at night. It really is individual, so find a pattern that works best for you.

Sleep to stay slim

Along with moving more and eating well, your other body clock mantra is to get a good night's sleep! Research studies have found that not getting enough sleep can upset your body clock's control over the hormones and chemical messengers that regulate hunger and metabolism, such as cortisol, growth hormone, insulin and leptin. One big effect is that the body becomes more resistant to insulin and cannot process blood sugar properly.

Studies at the University of Chicago have also found that sleep-deprived people feel more hungry, seeking out crisps and sweets rather than fruit or vegetables! The end result can be food cravings, weight gain, especially around the waist, and a higher risk of developing type 2 diabetes and a range of heart health problems.

So how much sleep do you need? Expert opinion varies, but it is thought that somewhere between seven and nine hours is optimal.

Trouble sleeping? Try these tips

■ Keep to regular times for going to bed and getting up
■ Move more every day
■ Cut down on stimulants like caffeine. You may need a six-hour gap between drinking a cup of coffee and going to sleep
■ Keep to sensible alcohol limits (see the guide on page 88)
■ Avoid exercise or stimulating activities near bedtime (sex is the exception!)
■ Avoid large or fatty meals near bedtime, but don't go to bed hungry either
■ Establish a calming routine; take a warm bath, keep the lights low and draw the curtains
■ Try to work through any problems or worries earlier in the day

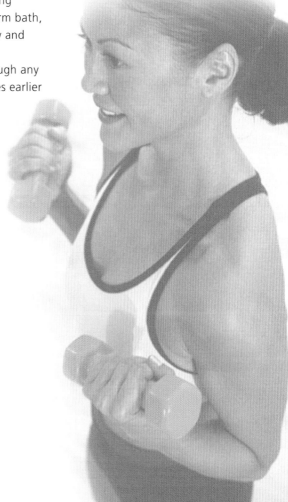

now just 'do it'

Hopefully, you are now convinced of all the benefits you get by eating regularly, moving more and getting enough sleep. So now it is time to actually do it! Healthy weight control is all about making changes that you can keep up, so the first step is to choose things you enjoy and that best fit into your daily routine. Then set yourself a start date.

To boost your well-being, take at least 30 minutes of moderate-intensity activity, five days a week (preferably daily). 'Moderate intensity' means brisk walking, gardening, cycling, dancing, walking up stairs, swimming, tennis, heavy housework like vacuuming, weight lifting – basically, any activity that makes you feel warm and breathe more heavily than usual. You should be able to carry on a conversation while doing the activity. If not, you need to slow down!

This 30 minutes or so can be done in one hit or in bursts over the day, and can be made up of different types of activities (see opposite).

Be active – burn calories

The body clock approach is designed to ease your body and mind into natural daily rhythms, helping your body to gently return to a healthier weight. Boosting your daily activity level to burn between 150 and 300 calories more than you currently do is an important part of it. This is equivalent to between 30 and 60 minutes of additional brisk walking over the day (or doing 10,000–15,000 steps in total – see page 29). As for all goals, it is vital to work out what is realistic and go from there.

This list tells you how long a 76-kg (12-stone) person needs to do different activities to burn 150 calories (double the time for 300 calories). Lighter people would burn a bit less, and heavier people a bit more for the same activity.

CALORIES BURNED BY DIFFERENT ACTIVITIES

Time taken to burn 150 calories (mins)

Activity	Time	Activity	Time	Activity	Time
Sitting quietly/watching TV	95	Table tennis	29	Gardening (digging)	15
Playing cards	80	Walking (briskly)	25	Walking uphill/up stairs	15
Standing	75	Golf	23	Aerobics (high intensity)	14
Ironing	60	Weight training (free weights)	23	Running – slow	
Painting (inside)	58	Aerobics (medium intensity)	20	(11 mins/mile; 7 mins/km)	14
Dancing (ballroom)	38	Badminton	20	Skipping	12
Gardening (raking)	35	Cycling (moderately)	20	Swimming (breast stroke)	12
Walking (average pace)	33	Dancing (modern)	20	Judo	10
Window cleaning	33	Horse-riding (trotting)	18	Running – rapid	
Cleaning	32	Scrubbing floors	18	(7 mins/mile; 4 mins/km)	10
Cycling (leisurely)	32	Tennis	18	Squash	9
		Swimming (freestyle, slow)	16		

Top 'move more' tips

■ Plan ahead and establish a regular routine, for example, be active at similar times each day

■ Start gently and build up gradually, week by week. Record your progress

■ Choose an activity you enjoy or make it part of something you have to do anyway, such as walking the dog, doing the shopping or the housework, using weights while watching television, taking the stairs, parking further away from your destination

■ Take any opportunity to walk more, and more briskly, and put more effort into your chores

■ Plan in your snack and a large glass of water one or two hours before you work out (see page 58)

■ If you go for the little and often option, every hour try doing something for a few minutes that makes you feel a bit breathless, for example, use weights (or baked bean cans or water bottles!), run up and down the stairs, do push-ups or sit-ups

■ Use an exercise bike in front of the television or listen to the radio or music as you walk

■ Arrange to be active with a friend or family member, or do something that involves other people

■ If you have children, plan activities over the weekend or in the evenings such as a family bike ride, walk in a park, rollerblading, dancing – this helps the kids develop healthy habits too

■ Remember to warm up properly before more intense exercise, especially first thing in the morning

■ Don't exercise if you are ill, and stop if you start to feel unwell. Check with your doctor first if you have any health problems or concerns

making the body clock diet work for you

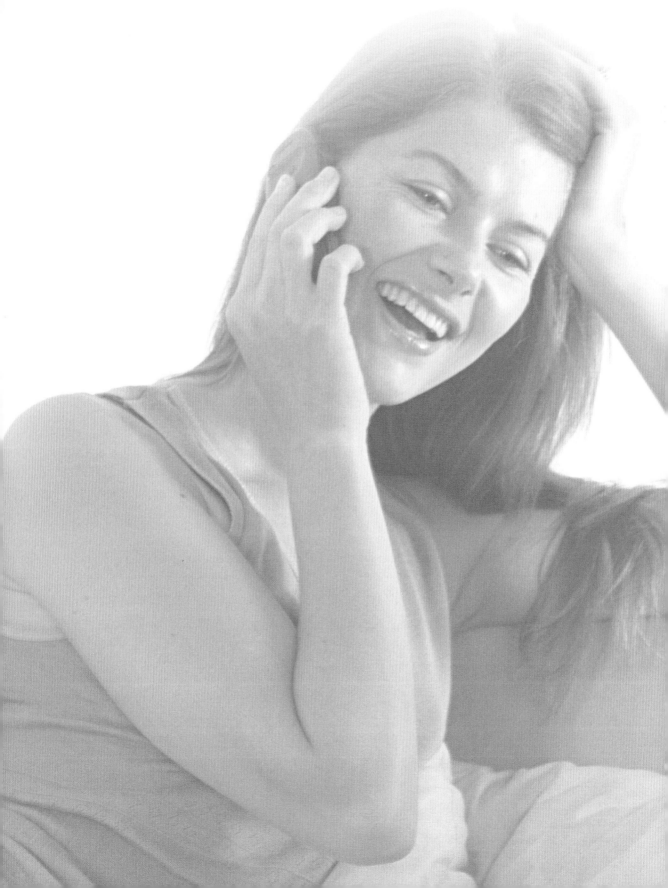

body clock questionnaires

Complete these two questionnaires to see how the body clock approach can work for you.

ARE YOU A LARK OR AN OWL?

1 When you have been up for half an hour on a normal working day, how do you feel?
A Very refreshed
B Fairly refreshed
C Fairly tired
D Not at all refreshed

2 How is your appetite after that first half an hour of being awake?
A Very good
B Fairly good
C Slightly good
D Not at all good

3 Suppose that you decide to exercise with a friend and the only time they can make it is from 7 am to 8 am. How do you think you would perform or feel?
A Would be on good form
B Would be on reasonable form
C Would find it difficult
D Would find it very difficult

4 At what time in the evening do you usually start feeling tired and ready for sleep?
A 8.00–9.30 pm
B 9.30–10.45 pm
C 10.45 pm–12.30 am
D 12.30–1.45 am
E 1.45–3.00 am

5 Suppose that you were able to choose your own working hours for a stimulating job. Which of the following three-hour blocks of time would be your most preferred work time?
A 4.00–7.00 am
B 7.00–10.00 am
C 11.00 am–2.00 pm
D 4.00–7.00 pm
E 9.00 pm–12.00 midnight

6 People often describe themselves as 'feeling best in the morning' or 'feeling best in the evening' types of people. Which do you consider yourself?
A Definitely a 'morning' type
B More a 'morning' than an 'evening' type
C More an 'evening' than a 'morning' type
D Definitely an 'evening' type

Scoring
Question 1: A = 7; B = 6; C = 4; D = 3
Question 2: A = 6; B = 5; C = 5; D = 4
Question 3: A = 7; B = 6; C = 4; D = 3
Question 4: A = 7; B = 6; C = 5; D = 4; E = 3
Question 5: A = 7; B = 6; C = 5; D = 4; E = 3
Question 6: A = 9; B = 7; C = 3; D = 1

Now find out if you are a lark or an owl
17 to 19 = Definite owl
20 to 23 = Moderate owl
24 to 29 = Intermediate – but more owl
30 = Intermediate
31 to 36 = Intermediate – but more lark
37 to 40 = Moderate lark
41 to 43 = Definite lark

Quiz adapted from: 'A self-assessment questionnaire to determine morningness–eveningness in human circadian rhythms' by Horne and Ostberg, 1976.

If you are intermediate, this is the most common category. You may have some preference for doing more in the morning or evening, but generally you will be flexible and fit comfortably with standard work times and sociable hours.

The more of a lark you are, the earlier you tend to wake and the better you feel in the morning; and the earlier you want to go to bed at night. It may help to plan your day and meals to run an hour or two earlier than most people, and do important things in the morning. You will suit work patterns that start and finish earlier than usual.

The more of an owl you are, the later you tend to wake and the better you feel in the evening; and the later you want to go to bed. It may help to plan your day and meals to run an hour or two later than most people, and do important things later in the day. You will suit work patterns that start and finish later than the usual working day.

WHAT ARE YOUR ATTITUDES TO LOSING WEIGHT?

Answer true or false to the following statements. (The positive responses are listed below.)

1 I have spent time thinking about my eating habits

2 I will only feel successful if I lose lots of weight

3 I want to lose weight for myself

4 I don't have time to plan ahead and often skip meals to try and lose weight

5 I feel ready to take the time to be more active

6 I have no control over my food cravings, especially before my period. If I see food I like, I simply have to eat it

7 I realize that losing weight won't solve other problems in my life

8 I hate eating breakfast and can't see the point of it

9 The only way I can cope with stress and worries is to eat

10 The only way to lose weight is to keep strictly to a diet at all times

11 Even though I am busy, I am aware that it is important to have regular sleep times

Now work out your score.

Give yourself one point if you answered 'true' to questions 1, 3, 5, 7 and 11.

Give yourself one point for answering 'false' to questions 2, 4, 6, 8, 9 and 10.

If you scored less than 5, then re-read this book carefully. Look back at the questions you did not give the positive response to (see below) and plan to tackle those particular issues. If you scored over 8, it indicates that you have a realistic approach to losing weight, and will find that the body clock diet's holistic approach will really help you to achieve lasting success.

1 True
2 False
3 True
4 False
5 True
6 False
7 True
8 False
9 False
10 False
11 True

what is a healthy weight for you?

You are reading the body clock diet because you want to lose weight and get the best from life. But do you need to lose weight for your health's sake? Despite the fact that two-thirds of adults are overweight, it is easy to get a distorted view of your own weight thanks to thin media images.

Trying to be thinner than your body is naturally comfortable with puts you at risk of food obsessions and becoming a victim of the diet–binge cycle as you constantly fight against your body's regulators and rhythms. It can also mean that you find it hard to like yourself, and that in turn makes it hard to look after yourself properly. We are all different shapes and sizes, and you have your unique personality that reflects the real you – something your stomach or thighs can't do, no matter how flat or toned they are.

If you find you don't need to or don't want to lose weight, then you can use the body clock approach to maintain your healthy weight (see page 48) – which can actually be a big achievement in itself these days.

Discover your healthy weight

There is no single 'ideal' weight for anybody, but there is a healthy range. The point is to find a weight where you feel comfortable by living healthily and seeing where you naturally 'settle'. Losing weight is not just about appearance – it is also about health, and being able to do more of the things you want to do (see page 10).

Remember, if you are obese it could take nine years off your lifespan, but the good news is that you don't need to lose a lot of weight to reap real benefits. Losing 5–10 per cent of your weight can boost and protect your health and general well-being, including mood and self-esteem.

The Body Mass Index

The Body Mass Index (BMI) is the internationally used way of finding out if your weight is putting your health at risk. Use the BMI height–weight chart opposite to see how you fare by finding the point where your weight and height meet. The example shown by the dotted line gives the BMI for someone who is 1.7 m (5 ft 7 in) tall and weighs 82 kg (181 lb). This BMI puts them at the top end of the overweight category.

Alternatively, you can calculate your BMI as follows: your weight (in kg) divided by your height (in metres) squared. For example, the BMI for someone who weighs 72 kg (159 lb) and is 1.64 m (5ft 5in) tall is: 72 divided by (1.64 x 1.64) = 26.8.

Now read about your BMI

■ Less than 18.5 – you are underweight and you may need to gain weight for your health's sake. Talk to your doctor if you have any concerns, or if you feel frightened about gaining weight

■ 18.5–24.9 – you are a healthy weight, so aim to stay in this range

■ 25–29.9 – you are overweight and you should aim to lose some weight for your health's sake, or at least prevent further weight gain

■ 30–35 – you are obese and your health is at risk. Losing weight will improve your health

■ More than 35 – you are very obese. You should visit your doctor for a health check as you may need extra help to manage your weight and health. This is especially important before taking up any new exercise

Please note that BMI is not as accurate for athletes or very muscled people (muscle weighs more than fat), as it can push them into a higher BMI category despite having a healthy level of body fat. It is also not accurate for women who are pregnant or breastfeeding, or people who are frail.

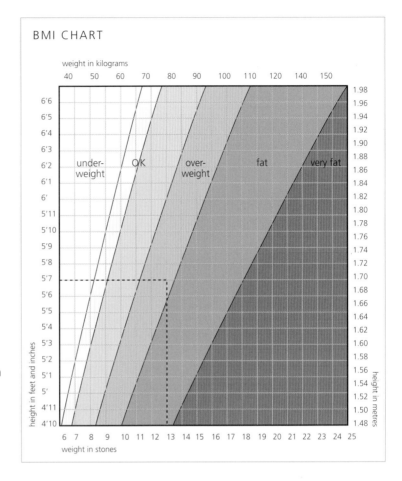

BMI CHART

Waist management

Another very important way to assess your weight is by measuring your waist at belly button level. It can be a better guide than BMI for men in particular, but everyone should try it.

■ For women, 81–89 cm (32–35 in) carries a risk similar to a BMI of 25–30; more than 89 cm (35 in) carries a risk similar to a BMI greater than 30

■ For men, the respective measurements are 94–102 cm (37–40 in), and more than 102 cm (40 in)

strategies for change

Before you start changing anything, take time to think about what you really want, and how you can best achieve your goals. Studies show that the more planning you do, the more likely you are to succeed. Planning also means you are far less likely to be thrown off course by a bad day, or the unachievable desire to look like a thin celebrity. This time you will be doing it for you, and learning to make great changes you can keep up, because you will feel so much more confident and in control.

Tips for getting started

Work out the pros and cons

When you make any change, there are always downsides (the cons) as well as upsides (the pros).

Write down what you see as the pros and cons of losing weight. For example, 'pros' could be looking better in my clothes and having more energy, while 'cons' could be not always eating what I want and making time for a daily walk. So do your pros outweigh your cons? If you are not sure, how would you feel if you were still this weight in six months'

time? Has that tipped the balance towards taking action?

Keep a diary

Keep a food, thoughts and activity diary to become more aware of your lifestyle habits. Research shows that those who use this strategy do best at losing weight. Carry a small notebook and jot things down over the day. List the time and what you ate, where you were, your mood and how hungry you were (if at all, see page 42). Also note any activity you do, and how much sleep you have. Be honest with yourself.

Identify barriers to losing weight

Use your diary to identify any real barriers or problem areas. Do you often eat when stressed or bored? Do food cravings ruin everything? Do you pick at food in the car or in front of the television? Do you nibble while you cook or prepare food? Do you skip breakfast or your exercise? Do you get enough sleep?

Get some support

A big part of your success will be having someone to take an interest and help keep you motivated. It could be a friend, partner, health professional, health club,

Internet 'buddy' or chat room. Remember, they are not mind readers, so let them know how they can help you most.

Setting goals

Losing weight is not all about willpower. Willpower is about deprivation and no one gets excited about that! Nor can anyone maintain it for long. Therefore, when making dietary changes, start small and set a few realistic goals – if the goals you set are achievable, you will then be able to stick with them and this will, in turn, increase your self-esteem and self-confidence. See page 79 for some ideas.

Decide what to aim for

Your overall aim is to eat well, move more and reach a healthier weight. As a guide, make your first weight goal to lose not more than 5–10 per cent of your weight – less if you prefer. For example, if you weigh 70 kg (11 stone), your first target might be to lose 5 per cent which is 3.5 kg (7¾ lb). Break it down into small steps, for example, around 2 kg (4½ lb) at a time.

Work out how to achieve your goals

The body clock diet includes meal plans to help ease your body clock and weight back on track. But long-term success requires long-term changes to all sorts of things, including the problems and barriers you identify in your food diary. Setting a goal should include a plan for how to achieve it, and how to overcome things that might get in the way. It helps if you make sure that your goals are SMART (see box right).

Track your success

Think how long it might take to achieve a specific goal and set a date to check it. When you achieve it, reward yourself with something non-edible. For example, a new CD, an item of clothing, seeing a movie, having a lie-in – whatever!

What to do if things go wrong

The first thing is not to panic. Ups and downs are a normal part of making changes. You are still learning new ways of doing things, and life's temptations are always there. For more information, see pages 43 and 45.

SMART GOALS ARE:

- *Specific*
- *Measurable*
- *Achievable*
- *Relevant*
- *Time-specific*

change your mind and your weight will follow

When you think about losing weight, what first comes to mind? Do you think of self-doubt and deprivation, or self-belief and positivity? If it is the former, your diet is doomed. If it is the latter, then you are well on your way to success. That is because how you think affects how you feel, and in turn the actions you take.

Coping with eating triggers

When you are surrounded by plentiful, tempting food, it is easy to eat when you are not actually hungry. Stress, boredom, coping with small children, the sight or smell of food, a party, giving up smoking, feeling upset, being alone or pure habit are all common eating triggers.

Often these triggers go way back to childhood, when we were given treats if we hurt ourselves, or to show love and attention. Triggers can become so automatic that you feel like you can't control what or when you eat.

Learning to tell the difference between true 'stomach' hunger rather than 'trigger' hunger will really help the body clock approach work for you. Try these tips:

■ Use your food diary to recognize if and when you are 'trigger' eating. Try to work out what you are really feeling, then look for ways you can change that feeling without using food

■ Keep to the body clock approach of regular meal and snack times

■ If you get the urge to eat after meals or snacks, talk to your urge. Tell it you know it is not really about stomach hunger as you have recently eaten. Distract yourself with another activity if need be, like going for a walk, calling a friend, changing tasks at work or drinking a glass of water. After 10–15 minutes, these urges or cravings tend to pass

■ If you are still not sure if you have stomach hunger, ask yourself before you eat 'I know I can have this food, but do I really feel like it or will I enjoy it?' You then have time to really choose, and so feel satisfied with your decision (and less likely to overeat), whatever it may be

■ Be inspired by knowing that each time you beat 'trigger hunger' you loosen its hold over you

Are you your harshest critic?

If you have had a bad day on the body clock diet, what are you likely to say to yourself? 'You are hopeless, you can't even follow simple meal plans, you may as well give up' or 'You've had a blow-out today, but overall you're doing well, and getting back to your regular eating is the key to staying on track'?

These automatic statements we make to ourselves are known as 'self-talk' and have a real influence on how we feel and act. Self-talk can be 'negative' and destructive or 'positive' and helpful. Try to stay on top of your self-talk. Your diary will help. When you find it getting negative, turn it around to the positive. That way positive actions, like keeping to your goals, will follow.

It was all going so well until ...

If those packets of crisps or chocolate biscuits are too hard to resist after work, or if you are a woman in your worst PMS moments (see page 80), don't feel guilty or tell yourself off. If you do, you are likely to think 'I've blown it now' and start bingeing, or worse still give up altogether. Instead, follow these steps to keep you on track:

■ Stop what you are doing and walk away from the food or the situation

■ Don't panic! Acknowledge that you have done well by stopping eating

■ Remind yourself that a lapse is normal and does not mean you have failed or that you have gained weight

■ If necessary, do something else to distract yourself

■ Think about what triggers led you into this situation and how you might deal with a similar situation next time

■ Have your next meal as planned. If you skip it, you will get hungry later and want to overeat again, throwing your body clock's appetite regulators out of sync and denting your confidence

staying on track

Once you are in the rhythm of regular meals and moving more each day, enjoying the body clock recipes and adapting your own favourites to fit the body clock way of eating (see page 54), your weight will start to come down. There are bound to be a few natural hiccups along the way, but you will soon learn to accept and deal with them rather than be thrown off course.

The longer you stay with your new rhythm, the better. While you can adjust your body clock's sleep/wake cycle within days, it can take a couple of months or so for the chemical messengers in your body and brain to reap the benefits.

As you lose weight, this process will be enhanced as your body adjusts to its new form. Insulin, a key hormone that influences appetite, blood sugar control and fat storage, will work more efficiently. Your regular sleep and exercise pattern will optimize the natural rhythms of your stress hormones and growth hormone, improving your ability to lose weight and burn fat.

You will be more in touch with natural 'stomach' hunger rather than 'trigger'

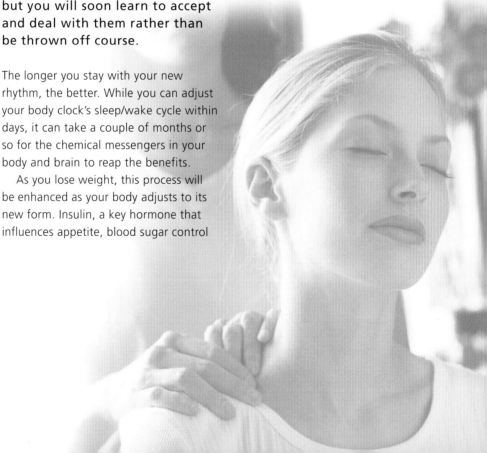

hunger, and regular meals will mean you avoid feeling so hungry that you end up bingeing. Old bad habits will become a thing of the past and new healthy habits will become the enjoyable norm – because you will feel so great! All this will also boost your confidence and reinforce your belief that you can control your weight, and it really is worth doing.

Don't expect instant results though. Learning new habits takes time. Think back to when you learned to ride a bike. No one expected you to do it first time. You no doubt had quite a few spills and needed picking up, with help along the way. Step by step you took control of that bike and learned how to keep it on course. Just like you will with your weight.

Tips to keep going

Life is never straightforward – there will be times when negative 'self-talk' creeps in to drag you back into old ways. It could be the lure of delicious food, a stressful period, feeling guilty, feeling fat, the upsets of shift work or hitting a dreaded weight plateau. So here are some tips to keep you going:
■ Value what you have achieved so far, rather than only focusing on what you plan to do
■ Look back at your 'pros' list about losing weight and refer to it often
■ Don't expect to change too much, too quickly – take things a step at a time
■ Remember to enjoy a non-food reward for achieving your goals
■ Use the body clock recipes and meal ideas to keep things interesting
■ No foods are forbidden on the body clock diet, and ups and downs are a normal part of change. If you have a bad day, forgive, forget and get back on track
■ Talk to your supporters and get plenty of encouragement – this is really vital!

Coping with a weight plateau

You have been steadily losing weight, then the scales start to stick. A few weeks go by and still no change, despite keeping to the body clock diet. What now? Maybe you need to spend time just getting used to your current weight, then deciding if you want to keep going. Fresh starts, when you feel ready, are motivating too.

Take another look at your portion sizes. Even slightly bigger portions add up over the day. This might explain why the scales are stuck! For example, look at what happens when you make a few changes to your meal plans:
■ A bagel rather than two slices of wholemeal bread – gain 70 calories
■ Three teaspoons butter on a bagel rather than two – gain 37 calories
■ 250 ml (8 fl oz) juice rather than 150 ml (¼ pint) – gain 40 calories
■ Tempted by crisps at the checkout – gain 185 calories
■ Six tablespoons rice with dinner rather than four – gain 100 calories
■ Large glass of wine rather than small – gain 85 calories

All these little extras result in an additional 512 calories over the day, which is enough to stop you losing 0.5 kg (1 lb) a week if it happens daily (see page 52). Keeping up with your food diary enables you to check portions and get back on track.

relax and nurture yourself slim

The body clock diet is not just about making the most of what you eat. It is a holistic guide to a healthier, confident and slimmer you. An important part of that is showing yourself the respect you deserve with proper rest and relaxation. If you often eat to cope with the stresses of life, taking care of yourself in this way is marvellous for replacing the comfort you once got from food. It helps keep your stress hormones and body clock in balance too.

Cleanse and relax

Busy lives, often dominated by the needs of others, can mean you rarely get time to think about how you like to relax or de-stress, let alone do it. But some 'me-time' is important, and a chance to clean out your 'mind toxins'. These could be anger, frustration, anxiety, poor body image and negative 'self-talk' (see page 43) – all ready and able to drain your energy and self-confidence.

Start by setting time aside to list what you would like to refresh in your life.

Your clothes? Your haircut? Your work? Your relationships? Your social life? When you decide, write down how you might do it, and when.

Try these mind-cleansing skills too:
■ When you're engaged in an everyday task, aim to devote 100 per cent of your concentration to it, whether it is washing the dishes, cooking or eating a meal or cleaning the car. Don't think about anything else, especially worries. This unbroken concentration helps to push aside anxieties, leaving you feeling refreshed and stronger
■ Look at yourself in the mirror, without your clothes, and note three things you like about any part of your body. Do this regularly, and increase your list
■ Feeling stressed or angry? Then let it out. Whether on paper, as a deep groan or hum, with a punch bag, a brisk walk or slow and regular breathing. Find a strategy that suits you. This will not only relieve the pressure, it also helps stop you taking your anger out on others, which can be upsetting all round – leading to guilt and more stress!
■ Imagine something you want to move away from (such as comfort eating,

negative self-talk or being a couch potato) and make the scene look grey and bleak. Now replace that picture with a bright, cheery, positive one of what you want to be doing instead

Plan – to relax

Spend five minutes at the end of your 'working' day to do these things, and start your next day feeling calm and centred:

■ If you work at a desk, clear and tidy it, file papers and contact numbers and save documents. If at home, do the same for kitchen work surfaces

■ Check your diary for tomorrow, list what you need to do and plan how each task will best fit in. Delegate anything you can

■ Think about your meals. What will you have? Will you need to take lunch with you? Is there anything you need to buy for the evening meal?

■ Plan in some 'me-time' – whether its 'moving more', a massage or reading time

■ Time your schedule to fit in best with any 'lark' or 'owl' body clock tendencies

■ Next day, keep to your list, and repeat the procedure at the end of your day

More ways to be nice to yourself

■ Have a relaxing bath
■ Book a massage or facial
■ Sit down and read your book or favourite magazine
■ Go to the hairdresser
■ Walk in the park on a sunny or invigoratingly cold day
■ Go to the theatre or cinema
■ Do some gardening
■ Visit a friend you have not seen for ages
■ Watch a favourite video/DVD
■ Buy yourself some new clothes
■ Apply a good fake tan
■ Sign up for an evening class

BEDROOM MAKEOVER

A good night's sleep is an essential part of the body clock approach. Combine it with some self-nurturing by making your bedroom a truly relaxing zone. Make sure you have a good mattress and curtains that make your room dark at night and open easily for a bright morning. Keep your haven for sleep and sex, not for work or other routine activities.

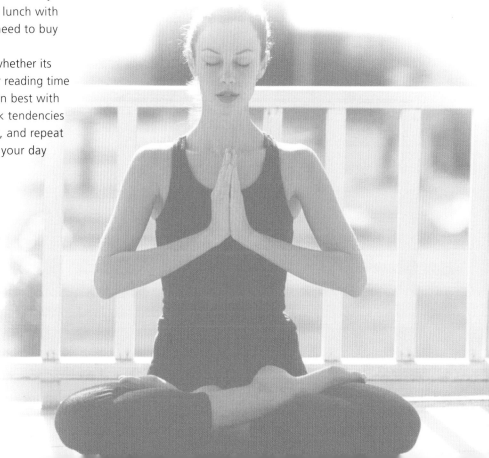

staying slimmer for life

Congratulations! You have achieved your healthier weight, you are in harmony with your body clock – and you are feeling great. And you will stay that way by keeping up your new-found attitudes, habits and motivation. Beware the trap of thinking 'Hurrah, I have lost weight, I can go back to my old ways!'

Now that you are slimmer, your body needs less fuel to keep your weight stable than it did before you lost weight. This is because there is now less of you to burn calories for energy (lighter people burn fewer calories than heavier people). Staying active will help off-set this a little, but you will still need to keep on eating differently.

That does not mean eating less food or going hungry, because the body clock way of eating is satisfying and allows plenty of healthy, filling foods. That is also why this book is not just a 'diet', but a guide to making lifestyle changes you can keep up. If you still find this hard to do, despite using body clock strategies, do talk to your doctor about getting some extra or specialist help.

Weight maintenance

If your weight has naturally stabilized, then that is great. If you have been losing around 0.5 kg (1 lb) a week, then keep up your regular body clock diet-inspired meals – plenty of fruit and vegetables, low-GI carbs, moderate amounts of protein (see page 53) – but have slightly more, say a bigger breakfast or lunch, or you may eat out a bit more often.

Take any changes slowly and step by step. Some trial and error is always involved to get the right balance. Keep a regular (at least weekly) check on your weight, waist size, body fat level or close-fitting item of clothing – whichever you prefer. Stay active and keep in contact with your supporters too. Research is clear that people who do are the ones who do best long term.

What do successful slimmers do?

An American study called the National Weight Control Registry investigated the habits of people who have lost at least 14 kg (30 lb) (for many it is 30 kg/66 lb) and kept it off for at least five years. It concluded that this is what they tend to do:

■ Always eat breakfast
■ Eat regular meals, and planned snacks
■ Continue to eat a balanced, low-fat diet
■ Regularly monitor what they eat, e.g. with a food diary or in their head
■ Stay more active, typically walking 4 miles (6.5 km) over the day, in addition to their usual daily routine (equivalent to a total of at least 15,000 steps)
■ Have a flexible approach to eating
■ Don't fall into the trap of feeling guilty about eating too much of a 'bad' food with the result of eating even more
■ Prepare most of their meals at home; occasionally eat out, but limit fast food
■ Watch portion sizes
■ Focus on what they have achieved, rather than yearn to be even slimmer
■ Cope with stress better
■ Regularly check their weight – at least once or twice a week, and get back on top of things if it increases by 2–3 kg (4–6 lb)
■ Realize they have to keep up their healthy changes for life

Maintaining your body rhythms

1 Stay aware of the ever-present food-filled environment and the power it can have
2 Stay realistic and be proud of who you are and what you have achieved; ignore fad diets and thin media images
3 Keep up your regular, healthy meals, moving more and making time for sleep and relaxation
4 Keep on consciously choosing what you eat, to stay in charge of 'trigger' hunger
5 Don't panic if you binge or gain some weight – forgive, forget and put your 'staying-on-track' skills into action
6 Make sure you have ongoing support
7 Enjoy the confidence and well-being boost that a healthier weight and being in control of food brings – it will help other areas of your life blossom too
8 Believe you are someone who can stay slim – and you will

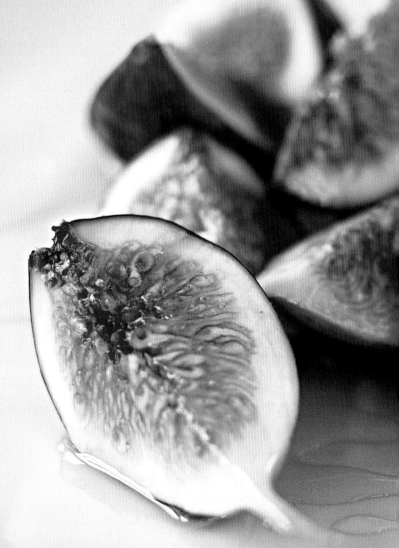

the
body clock
diet

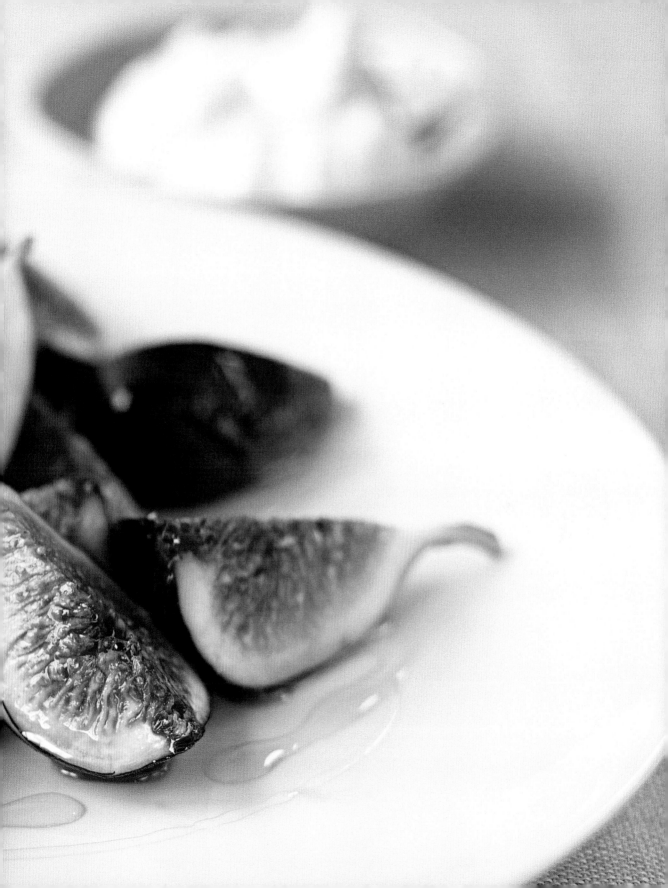

Getting started

Now to get going! Give yourself a definite start date for achieving your new healthier lifestyle. That includes taking advantage of the body clock diet's scrumptious and energizing meal plans. All these are nutritionally balanced and calorie-controlled to make life that much easier for you. And each day comes complete with daily tips and plenty of healthy living advice.

Regular meal plans will not only nourish your body, but help to optimize your blood sugar, appetite and energy levels at different times of the day – and so make weight control that much simpler. Combine these meals with plenty of moving more, more often, 'me-time' and a good night's sleep, and you will soon be in harmony with your bodily rhythms.

Nutritional know-how

The body clock meal plans have been carefully developed to provide what research suggests is an ideal balance of protein, healthy carbohydrates and fats. They include appetite-regulating low-GI foods (see page 23), bowel-friendly fibre and plenty of calcium; all are beneficial for weight control too.

Don't get too bogged down by counting calories. But it does help to know you need to take in around 500 calories fewer than your daily calorie needs to lose 0.5 kg (1 lb) per week. You can lose more if you are also more active, but a healthy weight loss is no more than 0.5–1 kg (1–2 lb) a week.

Each daily meal plan provides around 1,500 calories (which includes 200 ml milk for use in drinks such as tea, coffee and so on) – a level at which most women (who need to) will lose weight steadily (see pages 54–55 for how to adapt meal plans for men). You can mix and match breakfasts, lunches, evening meals and snacks from different days, or swap lunch for your evening meal if that suits you better. Pages 54–55 have advice on how to make your own meal plans, or make individual adjustments, body clock style.

Ten Dietary Commandments – eating the body clock way

1 Enjoy your meals and snacks at regular times each day – sit down, eat slowly and really taste your meals

2 Consciously choose what you eat; include some favourite foods or drinks and enjoy them without feeling guilty

3 Eat at least five portions of fruit and vegetables every day and choose wholegrain breads and cereals

4 Include a moderate portion of protein at each meal, e.g. lean meat, chicken, fish, eggs, reduced-fat dairy foods, pulses, tofu, nuts or seeds

5 Your meal should consist of half vegetables or salad and a quarter each of protein foods and healthy carbs

6 Eat fish at least twice a week, and make at least one portion an oily fish

7 Include two to three daily servings of reduced-fat dairy foods (or calcium-fortified soya foods)

8 Include some pulses, nuts and seeds on at least four days of the week

9 Choose olive or rapeseed oils and spreads – use sparingly

10 Drink at least six to eight glasses of fluids, with no added sugar, each day

Plan ahead

Successful slimmers plan ahead. It is important to have the right foods to hand when you need them, as it is easy to slip back to old habits with tempting alternatives around. Planning extends to meals for the day (or week) ahead, shopping and ensuring suitable meals and snacks are at work – or in the car if on the move. Planning will also help you feel confident and in control (see page 41).

Shopping the body clock way

Stock your kitchen with the following basic ingredients. Clear out all the foods that were part of your old, non-nurturing lifestyle while you are at it!

The fridge and freezer

■ Skimmed or semi-skimmed milk
■ Low-fat natural and fruit yogurt
■ Olive or rapeseed oil-based spread
■ Eggs – standard or omega-3-enriched
■ Parmesan, feta and/or other strong-tasting cheese
■ Low-fat/light cream cheese
■ Fresh fruit and vegetables and herbs
■ Low-fat salad dressings
■ Fresh or frozen lean meat, chicken or fish
■ Frozen vegetables
■ Frozen berries
■ Low-fat ice cream or sorbet

The store cupboard

■ Canned beans and chickpeas
■ Canned tomatoes, sweetcorn, reduced-fat coconut milk
■ Canned fish (not in oil)
■ Canned fruit in fruit juice
■ Pasta and egg noodles
■ Lentils, basmati rice, bulgar, couscous
■ Nuts, seeds and dried fruit
■ Dried herbs and spices
■ Olive, rapeseed, peanut and sesame oils
■ Different vinegars, e.g. balsamic, raspberry, red or white wine vinegars
■ Soy, chilli and fish sauce, horseradish, mustard, olives, capers

STOCK UP

As part of your planning, prepare a stock of body clock snack ideas, such as:
■ *portion packs of fruit and nuts (see page 82)*
■ *spiced nuts (see page 74)*
■ *pitta crisps (see page 70)*
■ *mixed seeds and dates (see page 58)*
■ *crunchy chickpeas (see page 100)*

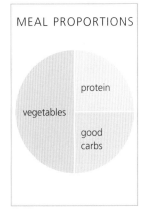

MEAL PROPORTIONS

protein

vegetables

good carbs

how to make your own meal plans – the body clock way

The body clock meal plans provide plenty of delicious recipes and ideas for healthy snacks. But you will also want the flexibility of creating your own. You can then mix and match them with ideas from this book to keep you on track with your healthy weight goals.

When planning meals and snacks, keep to the following servings from each food group every day to ensure your diet stays balanced and portion-controlled. Keep up your food diary too to monitor your progress.

IF YOU CHOOSE READY-PREPARED ITEMS

■ *Ready-made sandwiches or snack meals – choose one with around 300 calories*

■ *Ready meals – to have in place of a main meal. Choose meals with around 400 calories and serve with plenty of extra vegetables or salad*

SERVINGS PER DAY

■ Breads, cereals, potatoes, rice, pasta
Men 7–8 **Women** 5–6
■ Meat, fish, eggs, pulses, nuts
Men 2 **Women** 2
■ Vegetables
Men at least 3 **Women** at least 3
■ Fruit
Men 4 **Women** 3
■ Milk/dairy foods
Men 3 **Women** 3
■ Oils, dressings, spreads
Men 4 **Women** 3
■ Extras for snacks/drinks
Men 2 **Women** 1

What counts as a serving?

One serving of bread, potatoes, cereals, rice, pasta is:
■ A small bowl of wholegrain breakfast cereal or porridge
■ One medium slice of wholegrain bread, mini pitta or small tortilla
■ Half a medium pitta, tortilla wrap or roll
■ Three pure rye crispbreads or rice cakes, or two oatcakes
■ Two new or one medium-sized potato, half a jacket potato, 100 g (4 oz) sweet potato or six oven chips
■ Three heaped tablespoons (half a cup) of cooked pasta, egg noodles, couscous (25 g/1 oz uncooked)
■ Two heaped tablespoons (third of a cup) cooked rice or barley (25 g/1 oz uncooked)
■ Three heaped tablespoons beans, lentils or sweetcorn, or one corn on the cob
■ One level tablespoon nuts or seeds
■ Three cups of plain popcorn
■ One small slice of malt loaf, one digestive biscuit or half a scone

One serving of meat, chicken, fish, eggs, pulses, seeds and nuts is:
■ 75–100 g (3–4 oz) cooked lean beef, pork, lamb, chicken, turkey or oily fish
■ 150 g (6 oz) white fish or seafood

■ 150 g (6 oz) Bolognese sauce or chilli con carne
■ Two eggs (keep to about six a week)
■ Five tablespoons cooked beans, lentils, baked beans or tofu
■ Three tablespoons (35 g/1½ oz) nuts, seeds or hummus. Note: uncooked weights for meat, poultry and fish are 25–30 per cent bigger than cooked weights

One serving of vegetables is:
■ Three heaped tablespoons of any type – fresh, frozen or canned
■ A cereal bowl full of salad
■ One medium or seven cherry tomatoes or a portion of tomato sauce for pasta

One serving of fruit is:
■ One medium-sized fruit such as an apple, orange or pear
■ One cupful of berries or grapes
■ Two small fruits such as plums
■ A large slice of a large fruit such as melon or pineapple
■ Three tablespoons canned or stewed fruit in juice
■ 150 ml (¼ pint) fruit juice
■ One tablespoon dried fruit

One serving of milk and dairy foods is:
■ 300 ml (½ pint) skimmed or 200 ml (7 fl oz) semi-skimmed milk or soya milk
■ One small pot of low-fat natural yogurt, fromage frais or soya dessert
■ 25 g (1 oz) cheese
■ 50 g (2 oz) half-fat soft cheese
■ One small pot of cottage cheese

One serving of oil, dressing, spread is:
■ One teaspoon oil, spread, margarine, butter or mayonnaise
■ Two teaspoons low-fat spread or salad dressing
■ One tablespoon single or soured cream or half-fat crème fraîche
■ Two tablespoons fat-free dressing

Ideas for extras/snacks (around 100 calories)
■ Any two fruit servings
■ A small pot of low-fat yogurt or one other dairy serving
■ One slice of wholegrain bread with low-fat spread and yeast extract
■ Two crispbreads with 50 g (2 oz) tuna, thinly spread peanut butter or half-fat soft cheese
■ One crispbread with one level tablespoon hummus
■ One 25 g (1 oz) bag of nuts and raisins
■ One mini fruit bun, small cereal bar, mini chocolate bar or chocolate biscuit
■ A small bag of savoury snacks (around 100 calories)
■ A small glass of wine or 250 ml (½ pint) beer or cider or 25 ml (1 fl oz) liqueur

Drinks: use this drink guide every day
Choose at least six to eight drinks every day from the following list, totalling at least 1.5 litres (2½ pints).
■ Ginger infusion – add a little sliced fresh root ginger and a level teaspoon honey to a cup of boiling water; allow to infuse
■ Berry fizz – purée and sieve 75 g (3 oz) fresh raspberries or strawberries and top with 250 ml (8 fl oz) soda water
■ Tea or coffee (see page 27)
■ Water – tap, fizzy or still (see page 64)
■ Herbal or green tea

DO YOU HAVE DIFFERENT NEEDS?

■ *If you are male, or are very overweight or very active and losing weight too quickly (more than 1–1.5 kg/2–3 lb a week), then your calorie needs will be higher. You will therefore need to add one more serving from each of the following food groups: milk and dairy, bread and cereals, fruit and extras/snacks.*
■ *If you are losing less than 0.5 kg (1 lb) a week, despite being more active (assuming you can be) and following the meal plans carefully, try cutting back on one serving from each of the following food groups: bread and cereals, oils and spreads and fruit.*

day 1

Fuel up with an energy-recharging and sustaining breakfast based on slow-release carbohydrate such as wholegrain bread, with good-quality protein and a glass of fruit juice. Little and often will keep blood glucose, appetite and mood on an even keel, so plan ahead for your healthy snacks. Pack in some lunchtime protein to keep you alert in the afternoon and through the post-lunch dip. Then relax with a satisfying evening meal as your body prepares to slow down and sleep.

Breakfast

Small glass of cranberry juice
Slice of melon
1 thick slice of Granary toast with 1 tablespoon light cream cheese and 12 grilled cherry tomatoes
Tea, coffee or herbal tea

Snack

1 slice of malt loaf
Green tea or other herbal tea

Lunch

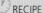 RECIPE
Chicken, grape and chicory salad with honey and mustard dressing
1 slice of crusty wholegrain bread
150 g (5 oz) low-fat fruit yogurt

Snack

2 tablespoons reduced-fat hummus
3 breadsticks

Evening Meal

RECIPE
Cajun-spiced swordfish with stir-fried vegetables
75 g (3 oz) steamed basmati rice

Exotic fruit salad
6 tablespoons apple juice
1 cardamom pod, crushed
1 star anise
150 g (5 oz) pineapple, mango and kiwifruit
1 teaspoon toasted shredded coconut

Bring the apple juice to the boil in a saucepan with the cardamom and star anise. Turn off the heat and leave for 10 minutes. Peel and slice the pineapple, mango and kiwifruit and place in a bowl. Pour the juice over the fruit and leave for a further 10 minutes. Top with the coconut.

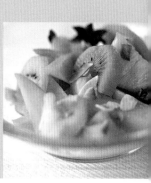

chicken, grape and chicory salad with honey and mustard dressing

Serves 1   Kcal 372   Protein 30 g   Carbs 48 g   Fat 8 g

100 g (3½ oz) cooked
   sliced chicken breast
75 g (3 oz) mixed black
   and green grapes,
   halved
1 head of chicory
1 handful of watercress

Honey and mustard dressing
1 teaspoon clear honey
½ teaspoon Dijon mustard
1 tablespoon light crème
   fraîche
black pepper

1   Put the chicken and grapes into a salad bowl. Separate the chicory into leaves and break the watercress into small sprigs. Toss the chicory and watercress with the chicken and grapes.

2   To make the dressing, put the honey, mustard and crème fraîche into a small bowl, season with pepper and whisk well.

3   To serve, pour the dressing over the salad and toss to mix thoroughly. Serve with a slice of bread.

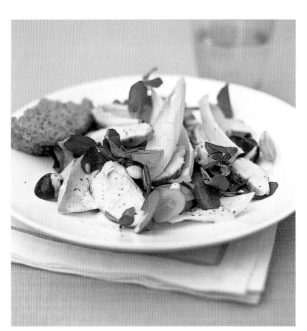

Cajun-spiced swordfish with stir-fried vegetables

Serves 1   Kcal 407   Protein 36 g   Carbs 40 g   Fat 13 g

1 swordfish steak, about
   150 g (5 oz)
1 teaspoon Cajun spice mix
1 teaspoon rapeseed oil
small piece of fresh root
   ginger, grated
1 garlic clove, crushed

300 g (10 oz) mixed
   vegetables, such as carrot,
   courgette, pak choi, sliced
2 spring onions, sliced
15 g (½ oz) unsalted
   cashew nuts
2 tablespoons oyster sauce

1   Rub the swordfish with the Cajun spice mix. Heat half the oil in a nonstick frying pan and fry the swordfish on each side for 2–3 minutes until cooked through. Remove from the pan and keep warm.

2   Heat the remaining oil in the pan and stir-fry the ginger and garlic for 1 minute, then add the mixed vegetables and stir-fry for 3–4 minutes. Stir in the spring onions, cashew nuts and oyster sauce.

3   Serve the swordfish with the vegetable stir-fry and basmati rice.

Five a day for health
All types of fruit and vegetables (except potatoes)
can count towards the recommended 'five a day',
whether fresh, frozen, dried, juiced or canned.
Eating five may be easier than you think.

Your body clock meal plans also include:
■ *200 ml (7 fl oz) semi-skimmed (or 300 ml/½ pint skimmed)*
milk for use in drinks, on cereal and so on. Or substitute for
a small pot of yogurt.
■ *If you would like a small glass of wine or a small beer with*
your evening meal, then replace dessert with a piece of fruit.

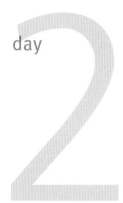

day

If you work out as part of your 'moving more' strategy, then make sure you are fuelled up. Exercising on an empty stomach makes you tire sooner, reducing how long and hard you train, as well as the amount of fat you burn. Make sure you have either a body clock meal two to four hours before, or a snack one to two hours before, to give your muscles the fuel they need.

Dehydration also causes fatigue. Have at least two glasses (200 ml/7 fl oz) of water two to three hours before exercising and use your water bottle during training. For some useful 'after work-out' tips, see page 70.

Breakfast	Small glass of grapefruit juice
	5 tablespoons wholewheat flaked cereal with dried fruit and 150 ml (1/4 pint) skimmed milk
	Tea, coffee or herbal tea

Snack	75 g (3 oz) dried mango, papaya and cranberry mix

Lunch   RECIPE

Grilled peppers with goats' cheese and butter beans
Slice of wholemeal bread
Piece of fruit

Snack	15 g (1/2 oz) toasted mixed pumpkin and sunflower seeds
	25 g (1 oz) chopped dried dates

Evening Meal   RECIPE

Chicken and butternut squash risotto

Fruit kebabs with strawberry sauce

200 g (7 oz) firm mixed fruit, such as strawberries, raspberries, nectarines and melon
2 tablespoons icing sugar
125 g (4 oz) strawberries
juice of 1 orange
2 tablespoons low-fat yogurt

Skewer the fruit on to kebab sticks – use whole berries and chunks of the other fruit. Spritz with a little water, then dust with the icing sugar and grill for 2–3 minutes under a preheated hot grill, turning occasionally. To make the sauce, in a food processor, whiz the strawberries with the orange juice until smooth. Serve with the yogurt.

grilled peppers with goats' cheese and butter beans

Serves 1   Kcal 350   Protein 17 g   Carbs 47 g   Fat 12 g

1 red pepper, halved, cored
 and deseeded
100 g (3¹/2 oz) canned
 flageolet beans, drained
 and rinsed
1 teaspoon olive oil
25 g (1 oz) firm goats'
 cheese

2 teaspoons pesto
To serve
25 g (1 oz) rocket leaves
drizzle of balsamic vinegar
drizzle of olive oil

1 Put the red pepper halves on to a baking sheet, skin-side down, and divide the flageolet beans between them. Drizzle with the oil. Cut the goats' cheese horizontally into 2 slices and arrange on top of the peppers. Top each one with 1 teaspoon pesto.

2 Cover the peppers with foil and bake in a preheated oven at 200°C/400°F/Gas Mark 6 for 20 minutes until the peppers are tender. Remove the foil and bake for a further 10 minutes.

3 Arrange the peppers on a bed of rocket leaves and drizzle with a little balsamic vinegar and olive oil. Serve with a slice of bread.

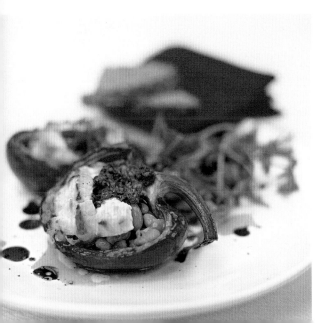

chicken and butternut squash risotto

Serves 1   Kcal 491   Protein 33 g   Carbs 53 g   Fat 17 g

1 teaspoon olive oil
1/2 small onion, finely
 chopped
300–450 ml (1/2–3/4 pint)
 vegetable or chicken
 stock
125 g (4 oz) butternut
 squash, peeled and cut
 into 1-cm (2.5-in) cubes

1 small boneless, skinless
 chicken breast, about
 125 g (4 oz), chopped
50 g (2 oz) risotto rice
1 tablespoon light cream
 cheese
1 teaspoon freshly grated
 Parmesan cheese
1 teaspoon chopped
 oregano

1 Heat the oil in a large saucepan and fry the onion until soft.

2 Meanwhile, bring the stock to a simmer in another saucepan.

3 Add the butternut squash and chicken breast to the onion and fry for 2 minutes. Then add the risotto rice and 1 ladleful of stock. When the stock has been absorbed, add another ladleful, stirring occasionally; continue adding the stock and simmering until the rice and squash are tender – about 20 minutes.

4 Stir in the cream cheese, Parmesan and oregano. Serve with a green salad or vegetables.

Seed storage
Once opened, seeds and nuts are best stored in a sealed container, preferably in the fridge, to keep them fresher for longer.

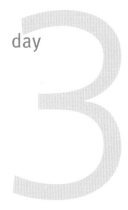

day

A little forward planning may be needed to cope with social situations. If you are going out to a restaurant for a meal, decide what you are going to eat before you leave. If you eat out regularly, it is unlikely to always be a treat. So opt for healthier choices and save the treats for true special occasions. If you are going to a party, have your meal or snack before you go – then stand away from nibbles and buffets. Useful tips for eating out include: skipping the bread and butter, asking for dressings and sauces to be served separately and avoiding pastry, deep-fried foods and rich desserts. See page 74 for tips on portion control.

Breakfast

Small glass of orange juice
1 chunk of soda bread with 1 teaspoon olive oil spread and 1 poached egg
Tea, coffee or herbal tea

Snack

25 g (1 oz) Japanese rice crackers with 2 tablespoons chilli dipping sauce

Lunch

 RECIPE

New potato, bean and avocado salad with mustard and cress
Piece of fruit

Snack

2 fresh plums
25 g (1 oz) crumbly cheese, e.g. Wensleydale

Evening Meal

RECIPE

Thyme-marinated lamb chops with aubergine and lentils
Green salad with a fat-free dressing

Frozen tropical fruit yogurt

100 g (3½ oz) frozen tropical fruit mix
100 g (3½ oz) Greek yogurt
1 passion fruit

In a food processor, whiz the frozen tropical fruit mix with the Greek yogurt. Place in a bowl, drizzle over the flesh of the passion fruit and serve straight away.

new potato, bean and avocado salad with mustard and cress

Serves 1   Kcal 350   Protein 7 g   Carbs 37 g   Fat 20 g

175 g (6 oz) cooked new
   potatoes, halved if large
75 g (3 oz) cooked green
   beans, halved
1 small avocado, sliced
1 handful of mustard and
   cress

Lemon yogurt dressing
grated rind and juice of
   1/2 lemon
1 tablespoon natural
   yogurt
1 tablespoon skimmed
   milk
few drops of Tabasco sauce
black pepper

1 Mix together the potatoes, green beans, half the avocado and the mustard and cress.

2 To make the dressing, blend the lemon juice and rind, yogurt, milk, the remaining avocado and a few drops of Tabasco sauce and season with pepper.

3 Drizzle half the dressing over the salad and toss well. The remaining dressing will keep for a day in the refrigerator, to use on another salad.

thyme-marinated lamb chops with aubergine and lentils

Serves 1   Kcal 490   Protein 42 g   Carbs 42 g   Fat 18 g

grated rind and juice of
   1 orange
1 teaspoon clear honey
1/2 teaspoon chopped
   thyme
2 lean lamb chops, about
   150 g (5 oz) in total
1 teaspoon olive oil

1 small onion, chopped
1 garlic clove, crushed
1/2 small aubergine, about
   125 g (4 oz), chopped
1/4 x 400 g (13 oz) can green
   lentils, drained and rinsed
2 tomatoes, chopped
black pepper

1 Mix together the orange rind and juice, honey and thyme in a large dish. Add the lamb chops, rub the marinade in well, then cover and refrigerate for 1 hour.

2 Remove the chops from the marinade and cook under a preheated hot grill for 4–5 minutes on each side.

3 Meanwhile, heat the oil in a nonstick frying pan and fry the onion and garlic for 3 minutes. Add the aubergine and cook for 5–6 minutes until browned and tender. Add the lentils, tomatoes and any remaining marinating liquid and stir well, then simmer for 2 minutes. Season with pepper.

4 Pile the aubergine mixture on a serving plate and arrange the chops on top. Serve with a green salad.

Stay positive
If you aren't losing weight as quickly as you would like to, stay positive and realistic. Focus on what you have achieved (and so feel successful), rather than the weight you still should lose (and so keep feeling a failure) and you will succeed.

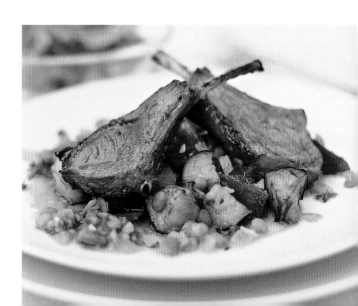

shift work case study

Shift work is common these days and could mean working through the night or doing regular or rotating shifts. Whichever time periods they cover, they have one thing in common: they make you work against the natural rhythms of your body clock. So at a time when your body clock dictates peak physical performance or concentration, you may be asleep. And when your body tries to wind down in order to rest and restore itself, you have to be at your most alert.

This wrestling between body clock and work patterns can take its toll on your health and sleep, and your weight. Then there are the social and relationship implications. You are going to work or just getting home when the family sits down for dinner or friends leave for a night out. It can be tough on all sorts of levels.

But on the positive side, shift work can suit some people. True 'larks' like nothing more than starting work early and being able to wind down in the early afternoon. And it will come as no surprise that 'owls' are more likely to be found working in bars or on evening shifts. But what if you are not an owl or a lark and have shifts to contend with? Here is Jan's story.

Jan is 38, married with three children and a senior nurse on a busy surgical ward. Over the years she has worked nights as well as rotating shifts. Jan loves her job, but working shifts on top of a busy life means that she now sleeps badly and has bowel problems and unhealthy eating (and drinking) habits. It's bad for her sex life too!

She often feels as though she has a 'tight elastic band around her head' and never wakes up feeling refreshed after sleep. Limited availability of food at work makes it all too easy to pick at chocolates and biscuits to keep her going through busy shifts, which is bad news for her waistline too.

Jan could not change her shifts, but she could change how she coped with them – and she reaped the benefits. The first step was to bring in a stock of fruit and healthy snacks for the week, and to spend an extra five minutes putting together a wholegrain sandwich, salad or low-fat ready-made meal for lunch.

To help her sleep, Jan invested in good ear plugs and 'black-out' curtains to make it easier to sleep during the day. She stopped her after-work wine 'night cap', as it made her wake to go to the toilet. She also tried to relax more on her days off rather than constantly rushing to do housework and chores – getting more support from her family really helped.

Top tips for shift work

■ Eat regular meals and planned snacks – body clock style – rather than pick throughout your shift. Have a mid-shift 'lunch' break, preferably with colleagues

■ Bring in healthy snacks such as fresh fruit, fruit scones, pots of yogurt or rice pudding, a flask of thick home-made vegetable soup, tuna salad snack pots, small packs of nuts and raisins, fruit salad, wholegrain cereal and carrots and celery with salsa or hummus dip

■ Caffeine can help keep you alert, but too much can interfere with sleep, digestion and mood – keep to no more than three cups of coffee or six cups of tea, and not near bedtime

■ Take a walk, change tasks or do some deep breathing if you begin either to feel tired or clumsy

■ Take naps during breaks, if time permits

■ To help you sleep during the day, drive home wearing sunglasses if it is bright, then ensure your bedroom is as dark and quiet as possible. Try wearing ear plugs and eye-shades

■ Stay as active as you can at work, including moving more

■ Think positive. If shift work is something you need or choose to do for now, then look at the pros as well as the cons. Talk to people who have established routines that work for them

■ Visit your occupational health staff for individual advice to ensure you look after your health the best you can

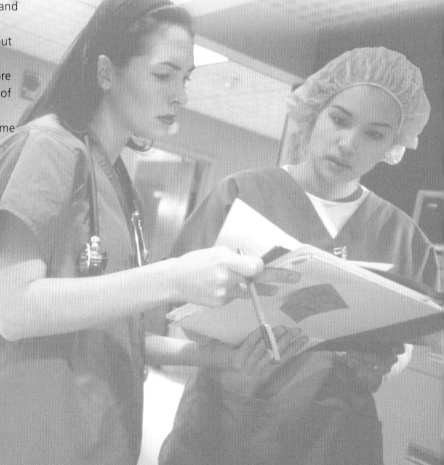

day **4**

The body clock meal plans give drink ideas (see page 55) to keep your body healthily hydrated. Around 60 per cent of your body is fluid, which is constantly lost when you sweat and breathe, and in urine and bowel motions. To replace it, you need to drink at least 1.5 litres (2½ pints or six to eight large glasses) of water or other drinks daily (see page 55) – more when it is hot and/or you are exercising (see pages 33 and 58) or you have had a big night out. Water is convenient and calorie-free. Drinking plenty helps fill you up and it also stops you confusing thirst with hunger.

Breakfast	Small glass of pineapple juice 2 slices of crusty wholemeal bread with 2 rashers of grilled bacon and 2 teaspoons maple syrup Tea, coffee or herbal tea
Snack	Pop 2 tablespoons popcorn in a little oil and sprinkle with a little chilli powder
Lunch	RECIPE **Speedy pizza** Green salad with a fat-free dressing 1 orange
Snack	200 ml (7 fl oz) semi-skimmed milk Piece of fruit
Evening Meal	RECIPE **Salmon fish cakes with mango salsa** **Lemon meringue crush**

Lemon meringue crush

1 meringue basket, roughly crushed
150 g (5 oz) natural yogurt
1 tablespoon lemon curd

Mix together the crushed meringue and natural yogurt until combined. Swirl in the lemon curd and serve in an attractive tall glass.

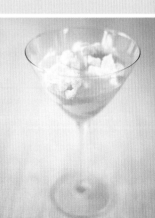

speedy pizza

Serves 1   Kcal 380   Protein 14 g   Carbs 73 g   Fat 6 g

1 large pitta bread
100 g (3¹/2 oz) new
   potatoes, boiled
   and sliced
2 spring onions, sliced
1 tablespoon light crème
   fraîche

15 g (1/2 oz) mozzarella
   cheese, chopped
1 tablespoon capers
salt and pepper

1   Split the pitta bread into 2 halves and place on a baking sheet.

2   Mix together the new potatoes and spring onions and arrange on top of the pittas.

3   Mix together the crème fraîche and mozzarella and spoon over the pittas, then sprinkle with the capers. Season well with salt and pepper.

4   Cook under a preheated hot grill for 2–3 minutes. Serve with a green salad.

salmon fish cakes with mango salsa

Serves 1   Kcal 449   Protein 22 g   Carbs 60 g   Fat 15 g

1 medium sweet potato,
   about 225 g (7¹/2 oz),
   peeled and diced
100 g (3¹/2 oz) salmon fillet,
   cooked and flaked
1/2 small red chilli, sliced
2 spring onions, sliced
1 tablespoon chopped
   coriander
plain flour, for dusting
1 teaspoon olive oil

salt and pepper
lime wedge, to serve
Mango salsa
1/2 mango, finely chopped
grated rind and juice of
   1/2 lime
25 g (1 oz) cucumber, finely
   chopped
1 tablespoon chopped
   coriander

1   Steam the sweet potato until tender. Drain and mash.

2   Put the sweet potato into a bowl, then stir in the flaked salmon, chilli, spring onions and coriander. Season well with salt and pepper. On a lightly floured surface, form the mixture into 2 fish cakes, then cover and chill for 30 minutes.

3   Heat the oil in a nonstick frying pan and fry the fish cakes for 3–4 minutes on each side until golden and piping hot. While the fish cakes are cooking, mix together all the salsa ingredients.

4   Serve the fish cakes with the salsa and a lime wedge. You can also make these with ordinary potatoes.

Avoid dehydration
To check whether you are drinking enough water, note the colour of your urine. If it is a light straw colour, that's fine; if it is dark, you need to drink more.

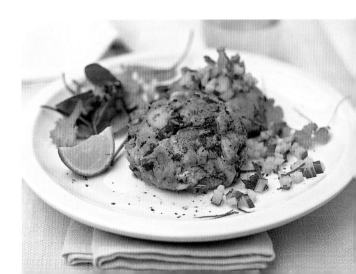

day 5

Today's meal plan features a warming, hearty vegetable soup that is quick to prepare. If you enjoy healthy soups, make them a regular feature of your ongoing body clock eating style.

French studies have found not only that daily soup consumers tend to be slimmer, but that the chunkier the soup, the more appetite-regulating it is. It seems that the bulky, low-calorie nature of low-fat soups ensures that the body's 'feel full' signals work optimally. So enjoy soup as a snack option, a starter or with wholegrain bread and fruit for a convenient and satisfying lunch.

Breakfast

Small glass of cranberry juice
150 g (5 oz) mushrooms sautéed in 1 teaspoon olive oil on 1 thick slice of Granary toast
3 fresh apricots
Tea, coffee or herbal tea

Snack

40 g (1½ oz) trail mix

Lunch

 RECIPE

Boston bean soup
1 slice of Granary or multigrain bread
150 g (5 oz) low-fat fruit yogurt

Snack

2 oatcakes topped with 1 teaspoon peanut butter and 1 teaspoon reduced-fat soft cheese

Evening Meal

 RECIPE

Baked trout parcels with low-fat tartare sauce
150 g (5 oz) new potatoes
Carrots and green beans

Baked banana

1 banana
15 g (½ oz) white chocolate, grated
1 teaspoon chopped hazelnuts
1 scoop of vanilla ice cream

Split the banana in half, sprinkle with the white chocolate, then sandwich back together. Wrap in foil and bake in a preheated oven at 200°C/400°F/Gas Mark 6 for 10 minutes. Remove the banana from the foil and put into a bowl, then scatter the hazelnuts over the top and serve with ice cream.

Boston bean soup

Serves 1   Kcal 413   Protein 17 g   Carbs 70 g   Fat 10 g

275 g (9 oz) can tomato
   soup
100 g (3½ oz) can baked
   beans (reduced sugar
   and salt)
dash of Worcestershire
   sauce

2 tablespoons canned
   sweetcorn kernels,
   drained
few drops of Tabasco
   sauce

1 Heat the tomato soup and baked beans in a
saucepan over a low heat until they start to simmer. Stir
occasionally so that they do not stick to the pan.

2 Add the Worcestershire sauce, sweetcorn and
Tabasco sauce to taste. Serve hot with bread.

Wholesome wholegrains

*Three or more daily servings of wholegrains can reduce
the risk of heart disease, certain cancers and type 2
diabetes by up to 30 per cent. A serving could be a slice
of wholegrain bread, bowl of porridge or wholegrain
cereal, three pure rye crackers or half a cup of brown rice
or wholewheat pasta – all body clock-friendly foods.*

baked trout parcels with low-fat tartare sauce

Serves 1   Kcal 283   Protein 33 g   Carbs 18 g   Fat 9 g

1 rainbow trout fillet, about
   150 g (5 oz)
grated rind and juice of
   1 lime
Tartare sauce
2 cocktail gherkins, finely
   chopped

1 teaspoon capers, roughly
   chopped
2 teaspoons light crème
   fraîche
1 spring onion, sliced
1 tablespoon chopped
   parsley

1 Put the trout fillet on a piece of foil and sprinkle with
half the lime rind and juice. Fold the foil into a parcel,
place on a baking sheet and bake in a preheated oven
at 200°C/400°F/Gas Mark 6 for 12–15 minutes.

2 Meanwhile, to make the tartare sauce, combine all
the ingredients in a small bowl and stir in the remaining
lime rind and juice.

3 Remove the foil and serve the trout with the tartare
sauce, potatoes and vegetables.

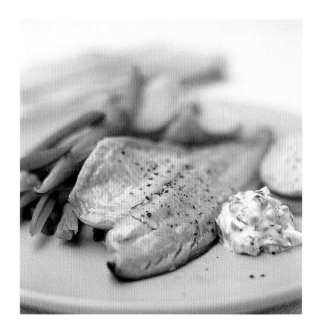

day

When you aren't having a body clock meal idea, here's how you can fit other foods or ready-made sandwiches and salads into your healthy eating plan. 'Guideline daily amounts' have been developed by health experts to help people see how a particular food type fits into a healthy diet, if they are maintaining their weight. These are listed opposite, along with corresponding values for the body clock diet.

Breakfast	Freshly squeezed juice of 3 oranges
	1 low-fat fruit yogurt with 1 banana, sliced
	Tea, coffee or herbal tea

Snack

12 olives
1 handful of cherry tomatoes
1 small breakfast muffin

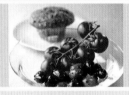

Lunch

 RECIPE

Chicken salad with peanut dressing
2 slices of toasted ciabatta
100 g (3½ oz) low-fat rice pudding

Snack

3 fresh dates with 2 tablespoons extra-light cream cheese

Evening Meal

 RECIPE

Prawn Laksa

Griddled pineapple with pistachio nuts

1 tablespoon dark rum
1 tablespoon muscovado sugar
2 slices of fresh or canned pineapple
1 tablespoon pistachio nuts, toasted
1 tablespoon natural yogurt

Mix together the rum and sugar. Spoon the sugar mixture over the pineapple. Heat a griddle or frying pan until hot and cook the pineapple for 2–3 minutes on each side until golden. Remove from the pan, put into a bowl and sprinkle with the pistachio nuts. Serve with the yogurt.

chicken salad with peanut dressing

Serves 1   Kcal 483   Protein 32 g   Carbs 47 g   Fat 10 g

65 g (2½ oz) salad leaves, washed and dried
100 g (3½ oz) cooked chicken breast, shredded
6 cherry tomatoes, halved
5-cm (½-in) piece of cucumber, diced

Peanut dressing
1 teaspoon crunchy peanut butter
1 teaspoon sweet chilli sauce
2 tablespoons coconut milk or skimmed milk

1 In a large bowl, mix together the salad leaves, chicken, cherry tomatoes and cucumber.

2 To make the dressing, in a small bowl, mix together all the dressing ingredients until smooth.

3 Drizzle the dressing over the salad and toss well. Serve with toasted ciabatta.

Seafood specials
Prawns and other seafood can be part of a heart-healthy diet as they are low in fat, provide some healthy omega-3 fats and in moderation don't raise cholesterol levels.

Guideline daily amounts				
	Men	**Men on diet**	**Women**	**Women on diet**
Calories	*2,500*	*2,000*	*2,000*	*1,500*
Fat (g)	*95*	*70*	*70*	*55*
of which saturates (g)	*30*	*20*	*20*	*17*
Sugar (g)	*70*	*50*	*50*	*38*
Salt/sodium (g)	*7/2.5*	*5/2.0*	*5/2.0*	*5/2.0*

prawn laksa

Serves 1   Kcal 272   Protein 18 g   Carbs 37 g   Fat 6 g

1 teaspoon olive oil
½ red pepper, cored, deseeded and sliced
100 g (3½ oz) mushrooms, sliced
1 teaspoon red or green Thai curry paste
150 ml (¼ pint) fish stock
150 ml (¼ pint) reduced-fat coconut milk

100 g (3½ oz) raw tiger prawns, peeled
2 spring onions, sliced
100 g (3½ oz) cooked rice noodles
1 tablespoon chopped coriander

1 Heat the oil in a medium saucepan, add the red pepper and mushrooms and fry for 3–4 minutes. Stir in the curry paste and fry for 1 minute. Pour in the stock and coconut milk and bring to the boil. Reduce the heat and simmer for 5 minutes.

2 Add the prawns, spring onions, rice noodles and coriander, stir to mix and cook for 2–3 minutes until the prawns have turned pink. You can make this recipe with cooked peeled prawns, in which case add them right at the end so they don't overcook but just heat through.

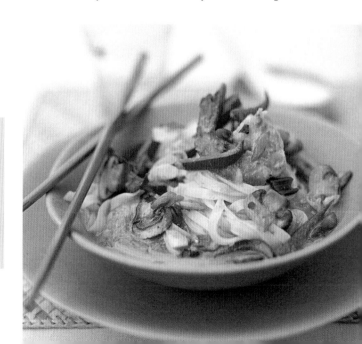

day 7

If you've worked out, well done! Now it is time to refuel your body ready for the day and night ahead. Your muscles' glycogen (carbohydrate) stores are optimally refilled, and muscles restored within the two hours after exercise, so if your next body clock meal is due within two hours, make sure you have it then. If not, have a body clock style snack instead – a smoothie, fruit and a glass of milk, pot of low-fat yogurt, small bowl of cereal or a couple of rice cakes with cottage cheese are all ideal. Be sure to drink plenty of water too.

Breakfast

Small glass of pineapple juice
125 g (4 oz) light Greek yogurt with 2 teaspoons clear honey and 1 tablespoon crunchy oat cereal
Tea, coffee or herbal tea

Snack

1 apple
25 g (1 oz) Cheddar cheese

Lunch

Heat a small can of minestrone soup and stir in 1 tablespoon pesto
2 slices of French bread with 15 g (1/2 oz) Grùyere cheese grilled on top
Slice of watermelon

Snack

🕐 RECIPE
Rosemary pitta crisps with tomato salsa

Evening Meal

🕐 RECIPE
Polenta-crusted pork with parsnip mash
Steamed Savoy cabbage

Ice cream with apricot purée

6 ready-to-eat dried apricots
grated rind and juice of 2 oranges
1 scoop of vanilla ice cream

Put the apricots and the orange rind and juice into a small saucepan and simmer over a medium heat for 5 minutes. Leave to cool slightly, then blend in a food processor until smooth. Serve with ice cream, and a little orange liqueur, if you like.

rosemary pitta crisps with tomato salsa

Serves 1 Kcal 159 Protein 4 g Carbs 29 g Fat 4 g

1 small pitta bread
1 tablespoon olive oil
1 teaspoon chopped
  rosemary
pinch of rock salt

Tomato Salsa
50 g (2 oz) tomatoes,
  chopped
1/2 red onion, finely
  chopped
1/4 red chilli, finely
  chopped
a little chopped coriander

1 Tear the pitta bread into bite-sized pieces.

2 In a bowl, mix together the oil, rosemary and rock salt. Toss the pitta bread in the oil mix.

3 Place the pitta breads on a baking sheet and bake in a preheated oven at 200°C/400°F/Gas Mark 6 for 10–12 minutes until golden and crisp.

4 Meanwhile, to make the salsa, combine all the ingredients in a bowl. Serve with the pitta crisps.

polenta-crusted pork with parsnip mash

Serves 1 Kcal 340 Protein 30 g Carbs 20 g Fat 16 g

1 small lean boneless pork
  chop, about 125 g (4 oz)
1 teaspoon seasoned flour
a little beaten egg
2 tablespoons instant
  polenta
1 tablespoon freshly grated
  Parmesan cheese
1 teaspoon rapeseed oil

2 parsnips, chopped
1 garlic clove, peeled
1 teaspoon chopped thyme
15 g (1/2 oz) butter or
  polyunsaturated
  margarine
black pepper
lemon wedges, to garnish

1 Toss the pork chop in the seasoned flour, then dip it in the beaten egg. Mix together the polenta and Parmesan and use to coat the chop.

2 Heat the oil in a nonstick frying pan and cook the chop for 5–6 minutes on each side until cooked through.

3 Meanwhile, bring a saucepan of water to the boil and cook the parsnips with the garlic for 12–15 minutes. Drain and mash with the thyme and butter or margarine, then season with plenty of pepper.

4 Garnish the pork with lemon wedges, and serve with the parsnip mash and Savoy cabbage.

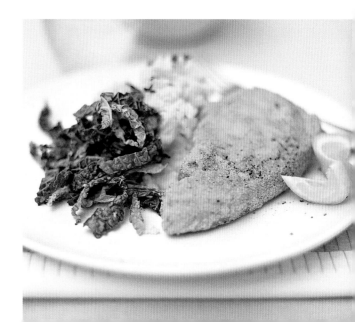

jet lag case study

Going on a long-distance flight is often exciting because it means 'holiday time'. Then again, it could be for the less-exciting prospect of work! Whatever the reason for the plane journey, travel causes two things: tiredness and jet lag.

Tiredness comes with the stress of preparation, sitting for many hours in less-than-spacious seats and dehydrating cabins and arriving in new places. Jet lag is the result of travelling across more than two or three time zones (the world is divided into 24 time zones), leaving your body clock no longer in sync with the time at your new destination.

For example, if you leave London at 10 pm, you could be in Sydney 24 hours later, but the time there is around 8 am. So your body clock says 'time for sleep', while Sydney says 'wake up and enjoy'! As a result, you are bound to feel tired, off your food, constipated and generally out of sorts.

Regardless of how far you travel, it is always a good idea to plan a restful first day to recover from the journey. The more time zones you cross, the longer it takes for the body clock to readjust – typically about a day for every two hours of time difference.

Everyone is different of course (and 'owls' seem to cope better than 'larks'), but adopting the local sleep, wake and eat patterns of your new destination as soon as you can will help you feel better quickly. New research from the University of Texas, Dallas, suggests that food as well as light can help to reset the body clock. Here is Nick's story.

Furniture importer Nick, 45, often travels from his home in London to Thailand and stays there for about five days. Getting away is always a rush and he is tired enough just from the hassle of sorting transport and hotels. Then there is the jet lag caused by the seven-hour time difference. He really needs a better approach.

Armed with body clock advice, before his next trip Nick checked that his passport, inoculations, visa, transport to and from the airport and hotel bookings were all in order a few days rather than a few hours before he left! On the flight he set his watch to Thai time and tried to sleep (it was night-time at his destination). He skipped the alcohol offered, kept to just one coffee and drank plenty of water and juices. He also brought along extra fruit to go with his meals, and walked about when he could.

When he arrived it was late morning, so rather than go straight to sleep, he went for a walk, then had some lunch. During the afternoon he swam and prepared for the next day's meeting – making sure he sat near light-filled windows. He had asked for an afternoon meeting since he would be more alert at that time of day.

Come bedtime, he wasn't really tired as his body clock told him it was only 4 pm. But he stayed in bed, blinds drawn, and rested until he finally dropped off. Next morning, although very groggy, he made sure he got up for his 8 am alarm call. After breakfast, a walk and a swim, he was the best he had ever felt at this stage of a trip.

If Nick was flying west, then he would basically do the opposite. He would need to delay rather than advance his body clock, since his destination time is behind his home time.

Tips for coping with jet lag

■ Be well prepared a few days before you depart
■ Leave plenty of time for travel to and from the airport
■ On the flight, set your watch to your destination's time and start living in line with it
■ Keep alcohol and caffeine to a minimum – drink water and diluted fruit juice instead
■ Eat light meals, and take some fruit to munch on
■ Adjust to your new destination's local times and routines as soon as you arrive
■ Keep to regular meal times, stay awake and be active and outside when it is light and sleep at night when it is dark

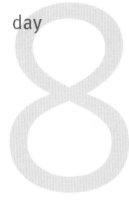

day **8**

When given a bigger portion, we eat more, but tend not to feel any fuller than if we had had a smaller portion, according to research from the University of Pennsylvania. So if you get used to large restaurant or fast-food portions, you are likely to serve large portions at home too.

As a guide when eating out, a healthy portion of rice or pasta looks like the size of your fist, and for meat or chicken the size of a deck of cards. If confronted with a big portion, decide how much you will eat before you start and leave the rest.

Breakfast

Small glass of grapefruit juice
Medium bowl of porridge with 3 fresh, canned or dried apricots
Tea, coffee or herbal tea

Snack

Vanilla smoothie
Whisk together 150 g (5 oz) vanilla yogurt with 200 ml (7 fl oz) skimmed milk and a few drops of vanilla essence

Lunch

Ciabatta with Parma Ham
2 thick slices of ciabatta
3 slices of Parma ham
15 g (1/2 oz) Parmesan cheese
8 cherry tomatoes, sliced
1 handful of watercress
1 teaspoon olive oil

Toast the ciabatta, then top both pieces of bread with the Parma ham, cherry tomatoes and watercress. Shave the Parmesan over the top and drizzle with the oil.

Snack

Spiced mixed nuts
1 teaspoon olive oil
pinch of rock salt
1/2 teaspoon paprika
200 g (7 oz) mixed nuts

In a small bowl, mix together the oil, rock salt and paprika. Toss the mixed nuts in the seasoned oil. Bake in a preheated oven at 200°C/400°F/Gas Mark 6 for 10–12 minutes, then leave to cool. Serve in 25 g (1 oz) portions.

Evening Meal

 RECIPE

Sticky chicken with lemon couscous
Steamed mangetout or asparagus

 RECIPE

Fruity baked apple

sticky chicken with lemon couscous

Serves 1   Kcal 400   Protein 26 g   Carbs 58 g   Fat 8 g

1 small boneless, skinless
  chicken breast, about
  125 g (4 oz), cut into strips
2 teaspoons clear honey
1 tablespoon soy sauce
1 tablespoon hoisin sauce
1 garlic clove, crushed
75 g (3 oz) couscous

250 ml (8 fl oz) boiling
  chicken stock
small knob of butter
2 spring onions, sliced
grated rind and juice of
  1/2 lemon
2 tablespoons chopped
  parsley

1 Put the chicken into a non-metallic bowl. In another bowl, mix together the honey, soy sauce, hoisin sauce and garlic and pour over the chicken. Cover and leave to marinate in the refrigerator for at least 30 minutes.

2 Remove the chicken from the marinade and put on a foil-lined baking sheet. Place under a preheated hot grill for 4–5 minutes, turning occasionally, until cooked through and beginning to char slightly.

3 Meanwhile, put the couscous into a heatproof bowl with the stock, butter, spring onions, lemon rind and juice and parsley. Cover with clingfilm and set aside for 5 minutes until the liquid is absorbed.

4 Fluff the couscous with a fork. Heat any remaining marinade, making sure that you boil it for 1 minute, and serve with the chicken and couscous. Also serve with steamed vegetables such as mangetout or asparagus.

fruity baked apple

Serves 1   Kcal 127   Protein 1 g   Carbs 32 g   Fat 0 g

1 large eating apple
25 g (1 oz) ready-to-eat
  dried fruit, such as
  cranberries, sultanas
  and apricots
1 teaspoon demerara
  sugar

1 Core the apple and score a line around the middle of the fruit.

2 Stuff the cored centre of the apple with the dried fruit. Sprinkle over the sugar and bake in a preheated oven at 200°C/400°F/Gas Mark 6 for 25 minutes until the apple is tender. Cut in half and serve.

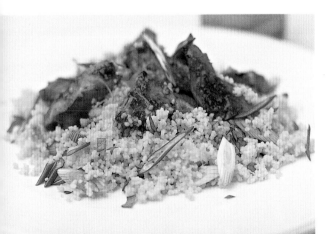

The bottom line
Half a kilogram (1 lb) of stored body fat contains 3,500 calories. So to lose that much in a week, a 500-calorie 'deficit' is needed daily (7 x 500 = 3,500). You can achieve this by consuming fewer calories or by being extremely active – or ideally by doing some of both; just like the body clock diet recommends.

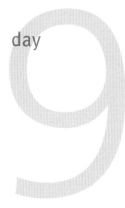

day 9

Eating planned snacks is a key part of the body clock approach to help keep blood sugar and appetite in check. If you sometimes find snacks hard to fit in, or feel like a bigger breakfast to get you through to lunch, then combine your mid-morning snack, like today's teacake, with breakfast, or have your mid-afternoon yogurt at lunchtime.

But do keep meal times regular, and make sure you have fruit to hand for an emergency snack, especially if you have a big gap between lunch and your evening meal. Three to four hours is the most you should go without a planned meal or snack

Breakfast	Small glass of fruit juice 2 fresh figs with 150 g (5 oz) low-fat natural yogurt and 1 teaspoon clear honey Tea, coffee or herbal tea

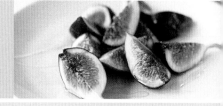

Snack	Toasted teacake with 2 teaspoons jam

Lunch   RECIPE

50 g (2 oz) mackerel pâté
1 medium pitta bread
Radishes and cornichons
Piece of fruit

Snack   150 g (5 oz) low-fat fruit yogurt

Evening Meal   RECIPE

Creamy chicken with pancetta and spinach
Steamed courgettes
175 g (6 oz) baked sweet potato

Blueberries and ice cream

125 g (4 oz) blueberries
1 scoop of vanilla ice cream

Heat the blueberries in a small saucepan over a low heat for 2–3 minutes until the juice begins to run. Transfer to a bowl and serve with ice cream.

mackerel pâté

Serves 1 Kcal 340 Protein 14 g Carbs 43 Fat 13 g

100 g (3½ oz) peppered
mackerel fillet
25 g (1 oz) light cream
cheese
1 tablespoon light crème
fraîche

1 teaspoon creamed
horseradish
2 tablespoons mixed
chopped herbs, such as
parsley, coriander and
lemon thyme
salt and pepper

1 In a food processor, blend together all the ingredients until smooth. Add salt and pepper to taste, then serve with pitta bread and radishes and cornichons.

Cook ahead
This pâté and many of the salad recipes are quick and easy to make either in the morning or the night before. This means they are ideal for a working lunch. Store in the fridge.

creamy chicken with pancetta and spinach

Serves 1 Kcal 397 Protein 40 g Carbs 32 g Fat 16 g

1 teaspoon olive oil
1 small boneless, skinless
chicken breast, about
100 g (3½ oz)
15 g (½ oz) pancetta, thinly
sliced
1 garlic clove, crushed
3 tablespoons chicken stock

1 tablespoon light crème
fraîche
1 handful of baby spinach
leaves
1 tablespoon freshly grated
Parmesan cheese
black pepper

1 Heat the oil in a large saucepan, add the chicken and pancetta and fry for 3–4 minutes, turning the chicken until it is browned all over. Add the garlic and fry for 1 minute. Pour over the stock, cover the pan and simmer for 10 minutes.

2 Stir in the crème fraîche, spinach and Parmesan and cook for 2–3 minutes until the spinach has wilted. Season with pepper and serve with steamed courgettes and baked sweet potato.

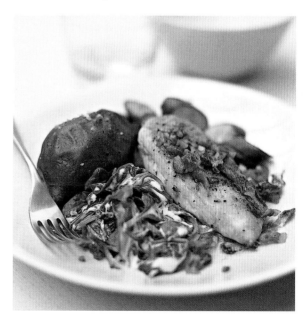

day **10**

Breakfast is a must for everyone, and especially on the body clock diet. It aids morning mood and concentration, and research from the University of Bristol, UK, found that people who ate a wholegrain breakfast cereal daily felt less fatigued, depressed and stressed.

Wholegrain cereals and breads gently raise blood glucose levels and re-stoke the brain's energy supply. They also provide B vitamins and other mood-influencing nutrients. Follow breakfast with regular meals and snacks that also contain a healthy balance of carbohydrates and protein to reduce swings in blood glucose and hormone levels – along with mood and food cravings.

| **Breakfast** | Small glass of orange juice
Slice of honeydew melon
4 tablespoons wholegrain cereal with milk
Tea, coffee or herbal tea |

| **Snack** | 1 pear |

Lunch   RECIPE

Pasta salad with crab, lemon and rocket
2 kiwifruit

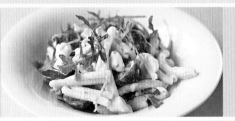

Snack   1 cheese scone

Evening Meal   RECIPE

Calves liver with leeks and cannellini beans
Green salad

Seriously chocolatey hot chocolate

200 ml (7 fl oz) skimmed milk
2 cardamom pods, split
25 g (1 oz) plain chocolate

Heat the milk in a small saucepan with the cardamom pods. Break the chocolate into pieces and add to the pan. Whisk until melted and smooth. Discard the cardamom pods and pour the chocolate drink into a mug.

pasta salad with crab, lemon and rocket

Serves 1 Kcal 330 Protein 22 g Carbs 49 g Fat 6 g

150 g (5 oz) dried pasta, such as rigatoni
grated rind and juice of 1/2 a lime
2 tablespoons light crème fraîche
1/2 x 170 g (51/2 oz) can crab meat, drained
8 cherry tomatoes, halved
1 handful of rocket leaves

1 Cook the pasta according to the packet instructions and leave to cool.

2 In a large bowl, mix together the lime rind and juice, crème fraîche and crab meat, then add the pasta and mix again.

3 Add the cherry tomatoes and rocket, toss together and serve.

Scoring goals
Try these 'SMART' goals (see page 41):
■ *When you get the urge to eat, stop and check if you really are hungry*
■ *Serve your meals on smaller plates*
■ *Eat without distraction of television or newspapers and pay attention to every bite*
■ *Don't keep tempting food in the house*
■ *Eat three planned meals and your planned snacks every day, starting with breakfast*
■ *Always sit down when you eat*

calves liver with leeks and cannellini beans

Serves 1 Kcal 389 Protein 39 g Carbs 39 g Fat 11 g

1 piece of calves liver, about 125 g (4 oz)
1 tablespoon seasoned flour
1 teaspoon olive oil
4 baby leeks or 1 large leek, sliced
1 rasher of lean back bacon, chopped
1/3 x 400 g (13 oz) can cannellini beans, drained and rinsed
1 tablespoon light crème fraîche
black pepper
1 tablespoon chopped parsley or thyme, to garnish

1 Toss the liver in the seasoned flour. Heat half the oil in a nonstick frying pan, add the liver and fry for 2 minutes on each side or until cooked to your liking. Remove from the pan and keep warm.

2 Heat the remaining oil in the frying pan, add the leeks and bacon and cook for 3–4 minutes. Stir in the cannellini beans and crème fraîche, season with pepper and heat through. Garnish with chopped parsley or thyme and serve with a green salad.

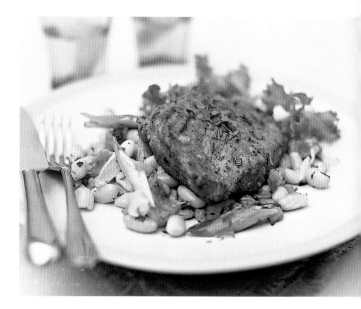

pre-menstrual syndrome (PMS) case study

Women's menstrual cycles are monthly body rhythms lasting around 28 days and are unique to women of child-bearing age. For some women they are regular and non-worrisome, but for others the mood changes and upsets they bring can sometimes take over their lives. Disturbances caused by stress, jet lag and lack of sleep can also throw menstrual cycles out of sync.

Most women are aware of some changes in their bodies and mood before their monthly period, and about one in three suffer some level of pre-menstrual syndrome (PMS). But for 1 in 20, it makes life a misery. PMS symptoms can start any time in the second half of the menstrual cycle and stop within two days of your period starting.

The causes of PMS are still unclear, but seem to involve fluctuations in hormones such as oestrogen and chemical messengers such as serotonin, both of which are connected to your body clock. The good news is that diet and lifestyle changes can make a difference. Here's Alice's story.

Just about every month Alice, 28, marketing consultant and mother, had five days of pre-menstrual misery. She felt irritable, tearful and less able to cope with everyday life. Then there was the bloating, food cravings and inevitable weight gain.

Fed up and determined to help herself, Alice contacted a national PMS society. They advised some fundamental changes to her daily diet to make it more regular and healthy.

After three months Alice felt much better. Eating regularly, having less caffeine and more fruit and vegetables really helped. She also liked the way she could have a little chocolate every day pre-menstrually if she wanted it – which satisfied her cravings without bingeing and weight worries. Alice now feels more in harmony with her body clock, and her relationship with food has improved. Most importantly, she feels more in charge of her body and well-being.

Carbs, serotonin and PMS

Cravings for sweet and carbohydrate-rich foods – especially chocolate – are common pre-menstrually. The finger of blame for this is often pointed at low levels of the chemical messenger serotonin, the theory being that the body tries to increase levels by making you eat more carbs.

More important, however, are the emotional responses to chocolate. You are unlikely to drive to the late-night garage to buy a packet of pasta, for example, but you would for chocolate because you want a food you love and associate with lifting your mood.

Nevertheless, you can blame low serotonin levels for something. Studies from the University of Leeds, UK, suggest that their true effect is to weaken control over appetite, making it that much easier to binge on desirable foods such as chocolate. The real problems start if you feel guilty and go on eating because you feel that your diet has failed.

Helping you through PMS

■ Keep a diary. Note when you menstruate, when you have symptoms and what they are. Keep it up to monitor improvements

■ Have three regular meals and two to three snacks, and ensure they contain slowly absorbed carbohydrate-rich foods (see pages 22–23) to help keep blood sugars, mood and cravings in check

■ Eat a balanced diet with five portions of fruit and vegetables daily, wholegrain breads and cereals, oily fish at least once a week – and limit caffeine, alcohol, salty foods and saturated fats (see pages 27 and 19)

■ Changes in metabolism mean that calorie needs can increase by around 200–250 calories a day. Build in an extra snack during your pre-menstrual days to appease cravings without guilt – this will reduce the risk of rebound bingeing

■ Take some daily exercise (see page 32) and leave time to relax (see page 46)

PMS snacks (200–250 calories)

Build one of these snacks into your usual daily meal plan to appease cravings:

■ Small (50 g/2 oz) chocolate bar or two bite-sized bars

■ A slice of cake or individual fruit pie or dessert

■ Three digestive biscuits

■ A bowl (50 g/2 oz) of favourite breakfast cereal with semi-skimmed milk

■ A fruit scone or fruit bun with 'light' white soft cheese

■ A 50 g (2 oz) bag of nuts and raisins

■ Two medium slices of bread with peanut butter or a little spread plus jam or honey

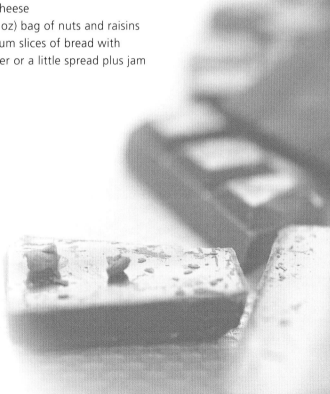

day 11

One important strategy successful slimmers use is to develop healthy cooking skills. This includes adapting long-standing family favourites rather than cooking new dishes all the time. Once you become familiar with which foods are better for you than others and what the right portion sizes are, then eating healthily will become automatic. A wholesome diet will no longer be a chore and you can really start to enjoy what you eat!

Breakfast	Small glass of chilled tomato juice Bagel with 1 slice of smoked salmon or wafer-thin honey roast ham and 2 tablespoons extra-light cream cheese Tea, coffee or herbal tea
Snack	**Vanilla smoothie** As before – see page 74. Add a selection of summer berries to this smoothie for a tasty change.
Lunch	🕐 RECIPE **Mixed grilled vegetables with a hummus dip** 150 g (5 oz) low-fat yogurt
Snack	15 g (1/2 oz) peanuts mixed with 25 g (1 oz) raisins
Evening Meal	🕐 RECIPE **Lamb and apricot tagine** 50 g (2 oz) prepared couscous

Roasted peaches

1 peach
grated rind and juice of
   1 orange
pinch of cinnamon
1 tablespoon quark

Cut the peach in half and put the 2 halves, skin-side down, into a small ovenproof dish. Mix together the orange rind and juice with the cinnamon and spoon over the peaches. Bake in a preheated oven at 200°C/400°F/Gas Mark 6 for 20 minutes or until tender. Serve with the peach juices from the dish and the quark.

mixed grilled vegetables with a hummus dip

Serves 1   Kcal 323   Protein 14 g   Carbs 42   Fat 12 g

375 g (12 oz) vegetables, such as aubergines, courgettes, onions and peppers
1 teaspoon olive oil
1 handful of basil leaves, roughly torn
50 g (2 oz) reduced-fat hummus

1 Slice the vegetables, place on a baking sheet and drizzle with the oil. Place under a preheated hot grill and cook for 12–15 minutes, turning the vegetables occasionally, until they are tender and beginning to char.

2 Scatter the basil leaves over the vegetables and serve hot with the hummus. These vegetables are also delicious prepared ahead and served cold.

Kick the habit
If you find yourself slipping back into bad habits, remind yourself about this well-known saying: 'If you keep doing what you have always done, you will keep getting what you have always got'. Ready for change now?

■ Trim meat of any fat, and remove the fatty skin from chicken; keep servings to around 90 g (3–4 oz)
■ Make meals healthy and satisfying with plenty of vegetables and salad
■ Use low-fat milks and fromage frais for sauces and toppings and to make mashed potato
■ Grill, bake, microwave, char-grill, stir-fry (using 1 teaspoon oil per person), poach or steam rather than fry

lamb and apricot tagine

Serves 1   Kcal 457   Protein 30 g   Carbs 50 g   Fat 17 g

1 teaspoon olive oil
100 g (3 1/2 oz) lean lamb, cubed
1 small onion, sliced
1 garlic clove, crushed
pinch of ground cinnamon
pinch of ground cumin
pinch of turmeric
200 ml (7 fl oz) lamb stock
50 g (2 oz) can chickpeas, drained and rinsed
3 ready-to-eat dried apricots
1 teaspoon toasted almonds
1 tablespoon chopped coriander
salt and pepper

1 Heat the oil in a medium-sized saucepan, add the lamb, onion and garlic and fry for 2 minutes. Stir in the cinnamon, cumin and turmeric and cook for a further minute. Pour in the stock and bring to the boil. Reduce the heat, cover the pan and simmer gently for 45 minutes.

2 Add the chickpeas and apricots and continue to simmer for 10 minutes until the lamb is tender. Stir in the almonds and coriander, season with salt and pepper and serve with couscous.

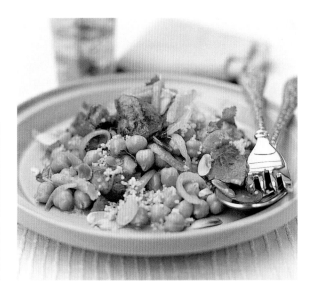

day 12

A simple way to get both balance and healthy proportions when serving up your meals is to divide your plate in half, then fill one half with salad or vegetables. Now divide the other half between protein-rich foods like meat, fish, eggs or beans, and carbohydrate-rich potatoes, rice, pasta, pulses, bread or noodles.

If you are having a combined dish such as tonight's pork meatballs with pasta, lasagne or a fish or shepherd's pie, then fill the protein and carbs half of your plate with that combination. Healthy eating couldn't be simpler!

Breakfast	Small glass of pineapple juice 3 tablespoons muesli with 100 ml (7 fl oz) skimmed milk Tea, coffee or herbal tea
Snack	1 pear
Lunch	RECIPE **Egg Florentine** 1 slice of wholemeal toast 1 handful of strawberries or a peach
Snack	25 g (1oz) Stilton cheese and 3 water biscuits

Evening Meal   RECIPE

Pork meatballs with fresh tomato and basil sauce

Shortbread with summer berries and quark

250 g (8 oz) berries, such as strawberries, raspberries and blueberries
1 tablespoon quark
2 shortbread fingers

Wash and prepare the berries. Place in a bowl and top with the quark. Serve with the shortbread fingers.

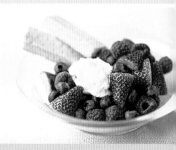

egg florentine

Serves 1   Kcal 295   Protein 13 g   Carbs 37 g   Fat 11 g

1 teaspoon olive oil
1/2 small onion, finely
   chopped
150 g (5 oz) frozen spinach
   leaves, defrosted

pinch of nutmeg
1 tablespoon light crème
   fraîche
1 egg

1 Heat the oil in a medium-sized nonstick frying pan and fry the onion for 3 minutes. Add the spinach and nutmeg and fry for a further 2–3 minutes, then stir in the crème fraîche.

2 Make a well in the centre of the spinach mixture. Crack in the egg and fry over a medium heat until the egg is cooked. Serve with a slice of wholemeal toast.

Steps to health

Don't forget lunchtime as a 'move more' time. Keep a pair of walking shoes at work and go for a walk during your break, if possible with a friend. This will help to recharge the brain cells for the afternoon and makes sure that the energy-draining post-lunch dip really is a thing of the past.

pork meatballs with fresh tomato and basil sauce

Serves 1   Kcal 485   Protein 31 g   Carbs 59 g   Fat 14 g

125 g (4 oz) lean minced
   pork
1 teaspoon pesto
pinch of dried chilli flakes
a little beaten egg
75 g (3 oz) dried pasta, such
   as fusilli or rigatoni

1 teaspoon olive oil
100 g (31/2 oz) cherry
   tomatoes, halved
1 handful of basil, torn
salt and pepper

1 In a bowl, mix together the minced pork, pesto and chilli flakes and season with salt and pepper. Stir through enough beaten egg to bind the mixture and form into 8 small balls.

2 Cook the pasta according to the packet instructions.

3 While the pasta is cooking, heat the oil in a nonstick frying pan and fry the meatballs for 4–5 minutes until browned and cooked through, turning them once.

4 Drain the pasta thoroughly. Toss with the tomatoes, basil and meatballs and serve immediately.

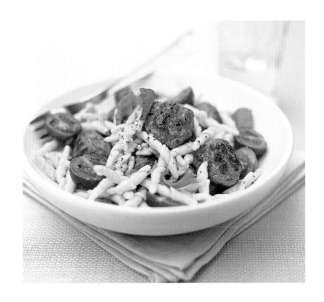

day

13

Weekends or days off are a time to relax and enjoy yourself, but that does not have to mean food overload. Rather than feel deprived of your past indulgences, use the flexibility the weekend brings to go out for walks, do something with the family, prepare and freeze healthy meals for the week ahead, go to the cinema or have an afternoon sleep or a massage.

If you eat out, save up some drinks and/or desserts from the week before to help balance your overall weekly calorie intake. This will help you to avoid overdoing it and gaining weight. If you do overdo it, don't panic. One blow-out won't ruin a week's good progress.

Breakfast

1 boiled egg
2 slices of Granary toast with 1 teaspoon olive oil spread and 1 teaspoon yeast extract
Tea, coffee or herbal tea

Snack

2 rice cakes with 2 tablespoons peppered cream cheese

Lunch

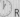 RECIPE

Grilled fresh sardines with tomato salsa
2–3 small slices of ciabatta
Piece of fruit

Snack

Fruit scone with 2 tablespoons quark and a handful of strawberries

Evening Meal

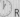 RECIPE

Peppered steak with crushed new potatoes
Tomato and red onion salad

Simple summer pudding

1 slice of day-old white bread
150 g (5 oz) frozen mixed berries
grated rind and juice of 1 orange
1 tablespoon icing sugar

Tear the bread into bite-sized pieces. Put the berries into a bowl and stir in the orange rind and juice, icing sugar and the bread. Set aside for at least 1 hour, for the fruit to defrost and the bread to soak up the juices, stirring occasionally. Serve with a little natural yogurt, or single cream as a special treat.

grilled fresh sardines with tomato salsa

Serves 1   Kcal 341   Protein 30 g   Carbs 27 g   Fat 13 g

2 fresh sardines, about
125 g (4 oz) in total,
cleaned
juice of 1 lemon
1 tablespoon chopped
parsley
salt and pepper

Tomato salsa
8 cherry tomatoes, chopped
1 spring onion, sliced
1 tablespoon chopped basil
1/2 red pepper, cored,
deseeded and chopped

1   To make the tomato salsa, simply combine together all the ingredients in a bowl.

2   Put the sardines on a baking sheet and drizzle with the lemon juice. Season with salt and pepper and grill for 3–4 minutes, turning once, until cooked. Sprinkle with chopped parsley and serve with the tomato salsa and toasted ciabatta.

peppered steak with crushed new potatoes

Serves 1   Kcal 350   Protein 42 g   Carbs 14 g   Fat 17 g

1 tablespoon crushed mixed
peppercorns
1 lean sirloin steak, about
150 g (5 oz)
150 g (5 oz) new potatoes
1 teaspoon olive oil

2 tablespoons light crème
fraîche
1 teaspoon creamed
horseradish
1 spring onion, sliced

1   Press the peppercorns into each side of the steak.

2   Cook the potatoes for 12–15 minutes until tender, then drain and keep warm.

3   Heat the oil in a nonstick frying pan and fry the steak for 2 minutes on each side or until done to your liking. Add half the crème fraîche and heat through.

4   Meanwhile, roughly crush the potatoes with a fork, then stir in the remainder of the crème fraîche, the horseradish and spring onion and mix well.

5   Serve the steak on a bed of the crushed potatoes with a tomato and red onion salad.

Gone fishing!
For your heart's (and mood's) sake, aim to have a serving of oily fish at least once a week – fresh tuna, or fresh, smoked or canned mackerel, salmon, pilchards, sardines, trout, swordfish or herring. All are good sources of omega-3 fats.

day **14**

Remember that good intentions dissolve in alcohol and drinking too much can upset body rhythms, add unwanted calories and slow weight loss. It is fine to continue to enjoy a drink, but most days have just the one. Above healthy limits – two to three units per day for women and three to four units for men – there is a continuously increasing risk to your health. A unit of alcohol (8 g by weight) is equivalent to:

■ half a pint (300 ml) of standard beer or cider
■ a small glass (125 ml/4 fl oz) of wine or champagne
■ a standard measure (25 ml/1 fl oz) of spirits
■ a glass (50 ml/2 fl oz) of sherry or port

Breakfast	1/2 pink grapefruit 2 level tablespoons no-added-sugar muesli topped with 125 g (5 oz) low-fat natural yogurt, 100 g (3 1/2 oz) chopped fresh fruit, such as apples, bananas and apricots Tea, coffee or herbal tea
Snack	**Mango and passion fruit smoothie** Blend the flesh of 1 mango with the juice of 1 orange and a handful of crushed ice, then stir through the flesh of 1 passion fruit.
Lunch	RECIPE **Tortillas** Green salad 1 orange Tea, coffee or mineral water

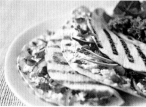

Snack	40 g (1 1/2 oz) pretzel crisps with 2 tablespoons tzatziki dip Ginger-infused tea
Evening Meal	RECIPE **Grilled haddock with lentils and spinach** Grilled tomatoes

Greek yogurt with summer berries and crushed amaretti biscuits

200 g (7 oz) mixed summer berries
4 tablespoons reduced-fat Greek yogurt
3 amaretti biscuits, crushed

Put the berries into a dish and top with the Greek yogurt. Sprinkle with the crushed amaretti biscuits, and a little demerara sugar if it isn't sweet enough.

tortillas

Serves 1   Kcal 250   Protein 12 g   Carbs 35 g   Fat 7 g

25 g (1 oz) ricotta cheese
1/2 red onion, finely sliced
1 tomato, finely chopped
1/4 green chilli, finely
  chopped
1 tablespoon chopped
  coriander
2 small flour tortillas
a little oil for brushing

1   Make a salsa by combining the ricotta cheese, red onion, tomato, green chilli and coriander in a bowl.

2   Brush the tortillas with a little oil, then cook very briefly on each side on a preheated hot griddle.

3   Spread half the salsa over one half of each tortilla, fold over the second half and serve with a green salad.

Easy does it!
Small changes can make a big difference. By having a mere 50 calories (one plain biscuit or half a glass of wine) less each day, you could lose 2.5 kg (5½ lb) in a year. Unfortunately, the opposite is true for gaining 2.5 kg (5½ lb), so take care!

grilled haddock with lentils and spinach

Serves 1   Kcal 385   Protein 40 g   Carbs 40 g   Fat 8 g

1 teaspoon olive oil
1/2 onion, finely
  chopped
pinch of ground cumin
pinch of turmeric
pinch of dried chilli flakes
1/3 x 400 g (13 oz) can
  lentils, drained and rinsed
75 g (3 oz) baby spinach
  leaves
2 tablespoons light crème
  fraîche
1 piece of boneless, skinless
  haddock, about
  125 g (4 oz)
lemon wedge, to garnish

1   Heat half the oil in a nonstick frying pan, add the onion and fry for 3–4 minutes until softened. Add the cumin, turmeric and chilli flakes and fry for a further 1 minute. Add the lentils, spinach and crème fraîche and cook gently for 3 minutes until the spinach has wilted.

2   Meanwhile, brush the haddock on each side with the remaining oil. Put the haddock on a nonstick baking sheet and cook under a preheated hot grill for 2–3 minutes on each side until done. Arrange the lentils and spinach on a plate and top with the haddock. Garnish with a lemon wedge and serve with grilled tomatoes.

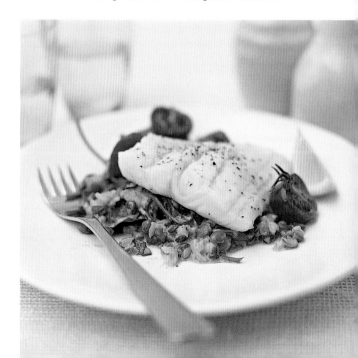

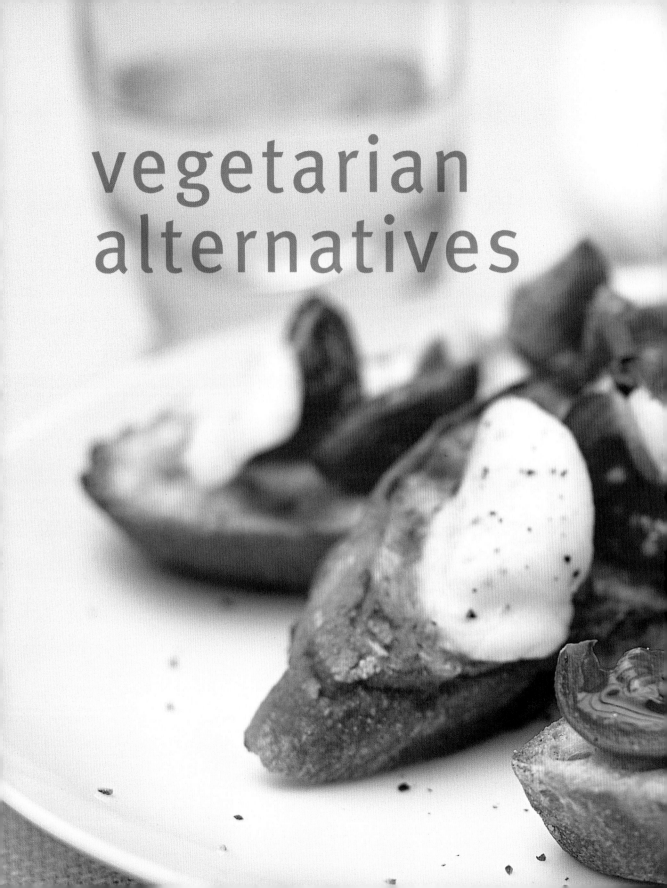

vegetarian alternatives

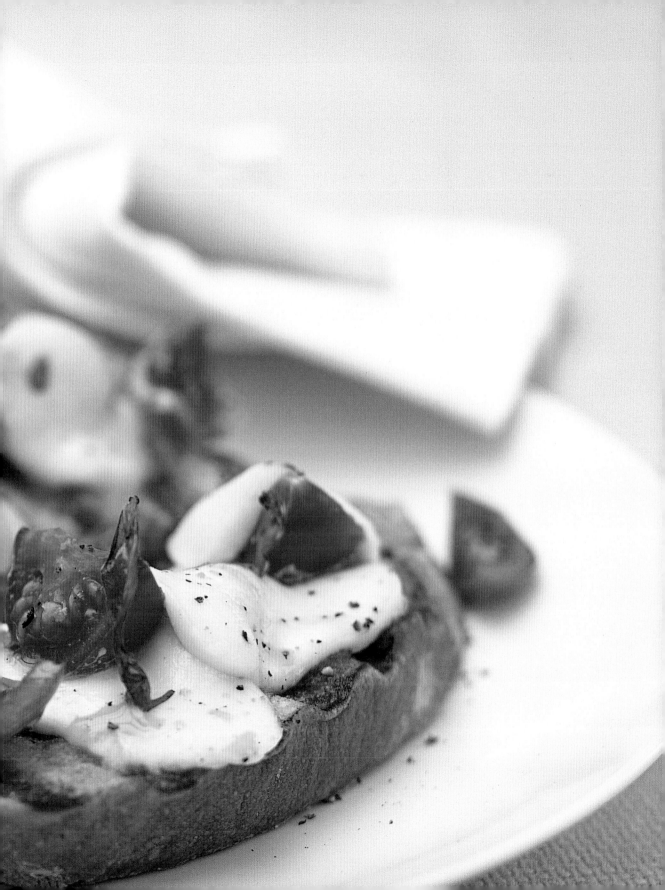

veg day 1

A healthy, balanced vegetarian diet includes foods from the main food groups (see pages 18–19). Remember that it is not enough to just cut out meat and eat more cheese, as they are from different food groups. Instead of meat and fish it is important to include nutritious protein-rich alternatives such as beans, lentils, tofu, nuts, seeds and eggs (if you eat them) in your daily diet.

Another 'must do' is to include good sources of omega-3 fats such as rapeseed oil and walnuts (see pages 19 and 25), since oily fish are usually the best source. If you also avoid dairy foods, see page 94.

Breakfast

Small glass of pineapple juice
1/2 grilled grapefruit
1 brioche or croissant with 2 teaspoons jam or marmalade
Tea, coffee or herbal tea

Snack

1 slice of malt loaf

Lunch

 RECIPE
Feta salad with low-fat dressing
150 g (5 oz) low-fat fruit yogurt

Snack

200 g (7 oz) mixed vegetable crudités, such as cucumber, carrot and peppers, served with 2 tablespoons reduced-fat hummus

Evening Meal

RECIPE
Thai vegetable curry
100 g (3 1/2 oz) steamed basmati rice

Summer berry jelly
1 packet blackcurrant or raspberry jelly
350 g (12 oz) mixed summer fruit, such as strawberries, raspberries and redcurrants

Make the jelly according to the packet instructions, then stir in the summer fruit. Transfer the jelly to a bowl and chill until set. This makes enough for 3 servings and can be kept in the refrigerator for up to 3 days.

feta salad with low-fat dressing

Serves **1**   Kcal 298   Protein 12 g   Carbs 50 g   Fat 6 g

1 Little Gem lettuce
25 g (1 oz) cucumber, chopped
2 tomatoes, chopped
1/4 red onion, sliced

25 g (1 oz) feta cheese, crumbled
2 mini pitta breads
1 tablespoon fat-free dressing

1 Wash and tear the lettuce into small pieces. In a large bowl, mix together the lettuce, cucumber, tomatoes, red onion and feta cheese.

2 Toast the pitta breads.

3 Transfer the salad to a plate, drizzle over the dressing and serve with the pitta breads.

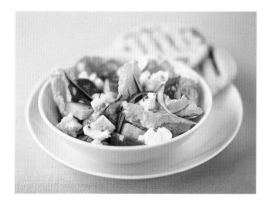

Rice as nice
Choose basmati or wild rice mixed with long-grain rice.
These varieties have a lower glycaemic index than other
types of rice, so can help you feel fuller for longer.

thai vegetable curry

Serves **1**   Kcal 498   Protein 12 g   Carbs 67 g   Fat 20 g

1 teaspoon oil
1 small onion, sliced
1 small green pepper, cored, deseeded and chopped
1 small red pepper, cored, deseeded and chopped
3 baby aubergines, halved, or 125 g (4 oz) large aubergine, chopped
3 baby courgettes, halved lengthways, or 1 medium courgette, chopped

75 g (3 oz) shiitake mushrooms
1 teaspoon green Thai curry paste
150 ml (1/4 pint) reduced-fat coconut milk
100 ml (31/2 fl oz) vegetable stock
1 tablespoon chopped coriander

1 Heat the oil in a nonstick frying pan, add the onion, peppers, aubergines, courgettes and mushrooms and fry for 5–6 minutes, stirring, until the vegetables are beginning to soften.

2 Stir in the curry paste and continue to fry for 1 minute. Pour in the coconut milk and stock and bring to the boil. Reduce the heat and simmer for 5 minutes. Stir through the chopped coriander and serve with rice.

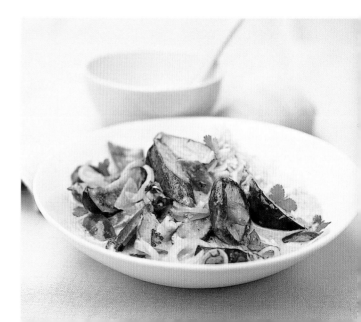

veg day

If you avoid dairy products, then it's vital to include other calcium-rich foods to help keep bones strong. Calcium aids weight control too. Dairy foods also provide a wide range of other nutrients, so the best alternatives are equivalent amounts of fortified soya milk and soya yogurt (see pages 18 and 55). Substitute these for dairy foods in body clock recipes. Use soya cheese too. Other good sources of calcium include calcium-fortified juice, canned sardines or pilchards, green leafy vegetables, pulses, bread, dried figs and almonds.

Breakfast	Small glass of cranberry juice 1 slice of panetone, toasted, served with 1 teaspoon olive oil spread and 2 teaspoons jam or marmalade

Snack

Dried fruit compote

100 g (3¹/2 oz) dried apricots, figs and prunes
150 ml (1/4 pint) Earl Grey tea
6 tablespoons apple juice
1 cinnamon stick
2 cloves

Place all the ingredients in a large saucepan. Bring to the boil, then remove from the heat and leave to stand for 30 minutes. Serve warm or cold.

Lunch

RECIPE

Baby spinach, walnut and blue cheese salad
300 g (10 oz) fresh fruit salad

Snack

Small cereal bar

Evening Meal

RECIPE

Leek and lentil filo tart
Mixed salad

Rice pudding with apricots and chocolate

200 g (7 oz) low-fat rice pudding
25 g (1 oz) chocolate
50 g (2 oz) ready-to-eat dried apricots, chopped

Warm the rice pudding over a low heat in a medium-sized saucepan. Chop up the chocolate and add to the rice pudding with the dried apricots. Serve hot.

baby spinach, walnut and blue cheese salad

Serves 1   Kcal 523   Protein 14 g   Carbs 80 g   Fat 18 g

100 g (3½ oz) baby
  spinach leaves
15 g (½ oz) walnuts,
  toasted
15 g (½ oz) Stilton cheese,
  crumbled
8 cherry tomatoes
1 pear, peeled, cored and
  sliced

Dressing
2 tablespoons apple juice
1 teaspoon clear honey
1 teaspoon wholegrain
  mustard
1 tablespoon chopped
  parsley
salt and pepper

1 To make the salad, in a large bowl, toss together the spinach, walnuts, Stilton, tomatoes and pear.

2 To make the dressing, mix together all the dressing ingredients and season to taste with salt and pepper.

3 Drizzle the dressing over the salad and serve with a hunk of Granary bread.

Iron absorption
Iron in non-meat foods such as beans, nuts, cereals and green vegetables is not as well absorbed as iron in meat. Boost absorption by having fruit, vegetables or juice that are rich in vitamin-C as part of the same meal.

leek and lentil filo tart

Serves 1   Kcal 375   Protein 24 g   Carbs 30 g   Fat 16 g

1 teaspoon rapeseed oil
3 baby leeks, finely sliced
¼ x 400 g (13 oz) can
  green lentils, drained
  and rinsed
25 g (1 oz) feta cheese,
  crumbled

1 egg
6 tablespoons milk, plus a
  little for brushing
6 x 15-cm (6-in) squares of
  filo pastry

1 Heat the oil in a nonstick frying pan and fry the leeks for 3–4 minutes until softened. Add the lentils and half the feta and stir into the leeks.

2 Blend together the remaining feta, the egg and the milk. Brush the filo squares with a little milk and use to line two 10-cm (4-in) fluted flan tins. Divide the leek mixture between the tins and pour over the egg mixture. Place the tins on a baking sheet and cook in a preheated oven at 200°C/400°F/Gas Mark 6 for 15–20 minutes until the filling is set. Serve with salad.

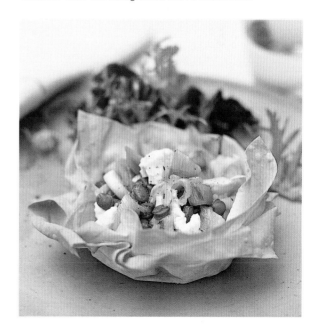

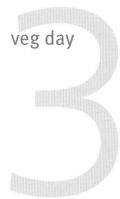

veg day

If you have skipped meals and eaten in an irregular pattern for a long time, starting to eat regular meals and snacks can feel a bit strange. But you will soon adapt, and once your regular eating puts you back in tune with your body clock and your appetite, you will feel more in control of what and how much you eat.

An American study of successful slimmers found that eating regular meals was one of their winning strategies. And it is a key part of advice for people recovering from binge-eating disorders, which often result in disruptions in the rhythms of hormones and other chemical messengers.

Breakfast	5 tablespoons wholewheat cereal with 200 ml (7 fl oz) semi-skimmed milk 1 slice of wholegrain toast with 1 teaspoon olive oil spread and 1 teaspoon jam or marmalade Tea, coffee or herbal tea
Snack	1 apple
Lunch	RECIPE **Omelette with rice, peppers, spring onions and sweetcorn** 200 g (7 oz) fruit salad
Snack	4 crispbreads with 2 tablespoons light cream cheese seasoned with plenty of black pepper
Evening Meal	RECIPE **Spaghetti with potato and beans and healthy home-made pesto** Mixed green salad **Caramel-style yogurt**

Caramel-style yogurt

150 g (5 oz) low-fat natural yogurt
1 tablespoon dark soft brown sugar
piece of fruit, such as apple, pear or banana

Pour the yogurt into a bowl and sprinkle the sugar over the top. Set aside for 10 minutes for the sugar to 'caramelize'. Serve with a piece of fruit.

omelette with rice, peppers, spring onions and sweetcorn

Serves 1   Kcal 303   Protein 11 g   Carbs 42 g   Fat 10 g

1 teaspoon olive oil
1/2 red pepper, cored, deseeded and sliced
3 spring onions, sliced
2 tablespoons sweetcorn kernels
75 g (3 oz) cooked mixed wild and long-grain rice
1 large egg
1 tablespoon chopped coriander

1   Heat the oil in a medium-sized nonstick frying pan. Fry the red pepper and spring onions for 2–3 minutes until softened, then stir in the sweetcorn and rice.

2   Whisk the egg in a bowl with the coriander. Pour the egg mixture into the frying pan and cook for 2 minutes, then place the pan under a preheated hot grill for a further 2 minutes until the egg is set.

spaghetti with potato and beans and healthy home-made pesto

Serves 1   Kcal 462   Protein 20 g   Carbs 77 g   Fat 10 g

75 g (3 oz) dried spaghetti
100 g (3 1/2 oz) new potatoes, sliced
75 g (3 oz) green beans, halved
Parmesan cheese shavings, to garnish

Pesto
1 small handful of basil leaves
1 teaspoon toasted pine nuts
1 teaspoon freshly grated Parmesan cheese
1 tablespoon natural yogurt
black pepper

1   Cook the spaghetti according to the packet instructions, adding the potatoes and beans 8 minutes before the end of the cooking time.

2   While the spaghetti is cooking, make the pesto. Put the basil, pine nuts, Parmesan and yogurt into a food processor. Season with pepper and whiz to a paste.

3   Drain the spaghetti thoroughly, then toss the pesto through it. Garnish with Parmesan shavings and serve with a salad.

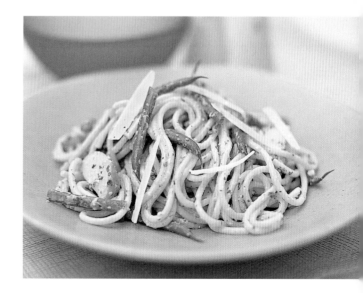

Being regular – it really works
Make sure you don't miss meals, even if you have eaten more than planned. Try not to let this 'unplanned' snacking happen often, otherwise it will interfere with your natural hunger development for the next meal – and slow your weight loss.

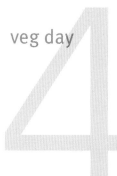

veg day

It's early days and you will still be getting used to things like better hunger regulation. Learning to tell the difference between true physical hunger and 'trigger' hunger (see page 42) takes time and practice too. A useful 'helper' is to assess and rank your level of hunger on a scale of 0–5 (0 = totally full, 5 = very hungry) before you eat.

When you eat for true hunger, you gain much more positive and conscious control over what and how much you eat. You will also feel satisfied and find it easier to meet your goals.

Breakfast	**Banana and yogurt smoothie**	
	1 ripe banana 150 g (5 oz) low-fat natural or vanilla yogurt 200 ml (7 fl oz) skimmed milk cinnamon, to decorate Tea, coffee or herbal tea	Slice the banana, keeping 2–3 slices for decoration. Place in a food processor, add the yogurt and milk and blend until smooth. Pour into a tall glass, scatter over the slices of banana and sprinkle with cinnamon.

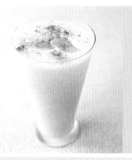

Snack	2 crispbreads with 1 tablespoon light herb and garlic cream cheese

Lunch	RECIPE **Potato wedges and red peppers with yogurt and parsley dip**

Snack	4 tablespoons wholewheat cereal with dried fruit and 200 ml (7 fl oz) skimmed milk

Evening Meal	RECIPE **Chilli beans** 175 g (6 oz) steamed basmati rice Green salad with a fat-free dressing Small pot of light chocolate mousse with chopped banana and a spoonful of light crème fraîche.

potato wedges and red peppers with yogurt and parsley dip

Serves 1   Kcal 362   Protein 11 g   Carbs 71 g   Fat 5 g

1 potato, about 175 g (6 oz)
1 red pepper, cored, deseeded and sliced
1 teaspoon olive oil
paprika
rock salt

Yogurt and parsley dip
3 tablespoons light Greek yogurt
1 tablespoon chopped parsley
2 spring onions, chopped
1 garlic clove, crushed (optional)
salt and pepper

1 Cut the potato into 8 wedges and cook in lightly salted boiling water for 5 minutes. Drain the wedges thoroughly, then put them into a bowl with the sliced red pepper and toss with the oil. Sprinkle with paprika and rock salt.

2 Arrange the potato wedges and pepper slices on a baking sheet and cook under a preheated hot grill for 6–8 minutes, turning occasionally, until cooked.

3 Meanwhile, make the yogurt dip. Put the Greek yogurt, parsley, spring onions and garlic, if using, in a bowl. Season with salt and pepper and mix thoroughly.

4 Serve the potato wedges and pepper slices hot with the yogurt dip.

chilli beans

Serves 1   Kcal 459   Protein 17 g   Carbs 88 g   Fat 7 g

1 teaspoon olive oil
1 onion, finely chopped
1 small green pepper, chopped
1/2 green chilli, chopped
1/2 x 400 g (13 oz) can mixed beans, drained and rinsed

200 g (7 oz) can chopped tomatoes
150 ml (1/4 pint) vegetable stock
1 tablespoon tomato purée

1 Heat the oil in a large saucepan and fry the onion, green pepper and green chilli for 3–4 minutes until soft.

2 Add the beans, chopped tomatoes, stock and tomato purée to the saucepan. Bring to the boil, then reduce the heat and simmer for 10 minutes.

3 Serve the chilli beans with basmati rice and a salad.

Get in the groove
You need to do something 20 times for it to become a new habit. So don't give up at the first or second hurdle. It takes time and practice to get confident with new weight-control skills and establish them as life-long habits.

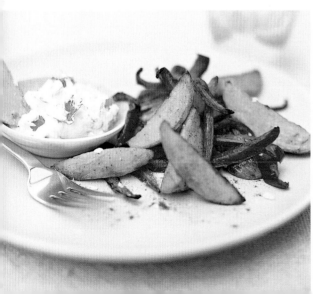

veg day

Vegetarians get most of their protein (see page 18) from nuts, seeds, beans, lentils, different grains such as wheat in bread and cereals, barley, rye, oats and quinoa, soya products, dairy foods and eggs. You may have heard of the need to balance the 'complementary' amino acids (building blocks of protein) in a vegetarian diet. This is much easier than it sounds. Eating a variety of vegetarian protein-rich foods each day, as found in the body clock meal plans, will provide the amino acids you require for good health. Protein-rich foods help to regulate appetite too.

Breakfast	Small glass of orange juice
	2 eggs scrambled with 1 tablespoon chopped fresh herbs and 1 tablespoon cream cheese
	1 slice of rye bread with 1 sliced tomato
	Tea, coffee or herbal tea

| **Snack** | Stir 2 chopped dried figs and 1 tablespoon clear honey into 150 g (5 oz) natural yogurt |

Lunch

Braised fennel with lemon and feta cheese

1 teaspoon olive oil	Heat the oil in a nonstick frying pan and fry the fennel for 1
1 fennel bulb, finely sliced	minute on each side. Pour over the grated lemon rind and juice,
grated rind and juice of	then add the stock and simmer for 5 minutes until tender.
1 lemon	Crumble the feta cheese over the top and season with black
2 tablespoons vegetable	pepper. Serve with a thick hunk of wholemeal bread.
stock	
25 g (1 oz) feta cheese	

Snack   RECIPE

Oven-baked crunchy chickpeas

Evening Meal   RECIPE

Marinated tofu with pak choi
175 g (6 oz) cooked rice noodles

Fresh strawberries with chocolate hazelnut spread

200 g (7 oz) strawberries	Wash, then quarter or halve the
2 tablespoons chocolate	strawberries. Serve with the
hazelnut spread	chocolate spread for dipping.

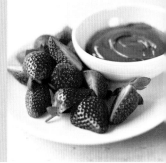

Oven-baked crunchy chickpeas

Serves 1   Kcal 141   Protein 7 g   Carbs 16 g   Fat 6 g

150 g (5 oz) canned
  chickpeas, drained and
  rinsed
1 teaspoon olive oil
pinch of rock salt

pinch of ground cumin
pinch of chilli powder
pinch of ground coriander

1 In a large bowl, mix together all the ingredients until they are well combined.

2 Place the chickpea mix on a baking sheet and bake in a preheated oven at 200°C/400°F/Gas Mark 6 for 10–15 minutes until golden. Allow to cool before serving.

Think positive

Make positive affirmations – inspiring statements about what is happening right there and then. For example, if your goal is to get back into a favourite pair of jeans, then your daily affirmation could be 'I am returning to the healthier weight when I could fit into the jeans I feel so great in.'

marinated tofu with pak choi

Serves 1   Kcal 379   Protein 15 g   Carbs 58 g   Fat 11 g

125 g (4 oz) firm tofu,
  cubed
1 garlic clove, crushed
1 teaspoon sesame oil
1 tablespoon soy sauce
1 red chilli, sliced

1 tablespoon chopped
  coriander
2 pak choi, quartered
  lengthways
3 spring onions, sliced

1 Put the tofu into a non-metallic bowl with the garlic, half the oil, the soy sauce, red chilli and coriander. Toss thoroughly, then cover and set aside for at least 30 minutes.

2 Heat the remaining oil in a nonstick frying pan. Remove the tofu from the marinade, reserving the marinade, add to the pan and stir-fry for 2 minutes. Add the pak choi and continue to stir-fry for 3–4 minutes, until the pak choi is tender. Add the reserved marinade and heat through. Serve with noodles.

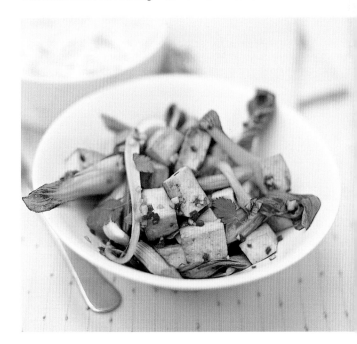

veg day

6

If you still find yourself saying things like 'I can't snack healthily when I'm in a rush' or 'I can't resist treats when shopping' or 'I must eat when watching TV', then stop, think and plan your positive solution. Believe that you are someone who 'can' do these sorts of things – and you will find a way. For example, you may decide not to leave home without an apple or cereal bar in your bag; only shop after you have eaten and with a shopping list; and make the TV room a food-free zone. Before long, these new habits will become the enjoyable norm.

Breakfast	Small glass of grapefruit juice 3 tablespoons muesli with 150 ml (1/4 pint) skimmed milk Tea, coffee or herbal tea
Snack	2 stuffed vine leaves, from the deli counter, about 75 g (3 oz) in total 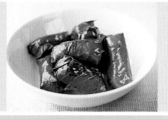
Lunch	RECIPE **Wild rice with feta, tomatoes, toasted seeds and oranges** Low-fat fruit mousse
Snack	200 ml (7 fl oz) semi-skimmed milk Piece of fruit
Evening Meal	RECIPE **Broccoli and pine nut pasta**

Rhubarb and custard

225 g (7 1/2 oz) fresh rhubarb
1 piece of stem ginger, finely chopped
1 tablespoon sugar
1 tablespoon water
4 tablespoons custard

Prepare and chop the rhubarb. Place the rhubarb, ginger, sugar and water in a saucepan and bring to the boil. Reduce the heat, cover and cook gently for 10 minutes, then leave to cool slightly. Pour into a dish and serve with the custard.

wild rice with feta, tomatoes, toasted seeds and oranges

Serves 1   Kcal 520   Protein 17 g   Carbs 85 g   Fat 15 g

150 g (5 oz) cooked mixed long-grain and wild rice
25 g (1 oz) feta cheese, crumbled
2 tomatoes, chopped

15 g (1/2 oz) toasted mixed seeds, such as pumpkin, sesame and sunflower
2 oranges

1 Put the rice, feta, tomatoes and seeds into a bowl and toss together.

2 Squeeze the juice from 1 orange into the bowl. Peel, then cut the second orange into segments, working over the salad bowl to catch any juice.

3 Put the orange segments into the salad bowl and toss to mix well. Serve straight away.

broccoli and pine nut pasta

Serves 1   Kcal 369   Protein 15 g   Carbs 50 g   Fat 13 g

100 g (31/2 oz) pasta
125 g (4 oz) broccoli, cut into small florets

15 g (1/2 oz) pine nuts, toasted
8 cherry tomatoes, halved

1 Cook the pasta according to the packet instructions, adding the broccoli 5 minutes before the end of the cooking time.

2 Drain the pasta and broccoli well, then add the pine nuts and cherry tomatoes. Toss well and serve while hot with a salad.

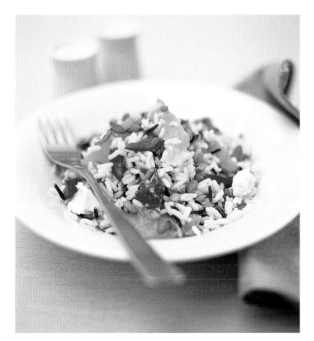

Snacks at work
Make sure you have body clock-style snacks to hand at work. Prepare suggested snacks ahead or keep a stock of ingredients in the kitchen or fridge. Easy standbys include fruit, pots of yogurt or rice pudding, cereal and milk, small cereal bars and small packs of dried fruit and nuts.

veg day 7

After playing a very difficult shot, a famous golfer was told by an onlooker 'You were lucky with that ball'. The golfer replied. 'It's a funny thing. The more I practise, the luckier I get'. The same can be said for other skills, including your new weight-control skills. In fact, an American study of successful slimmers found that those who had maintained their (realistic) weight loss for two to five years were far more likely to keep it off longer term. They weren't just lucky either. Their new skills and positive attitude had developed into an enjoyable way of life.

Breakfast

Small glass of cranberry juice
2 boiled eggs
1 slice of wholemeal toast with 1 teaspoon polyunsaturated margarine
Tea, coffee or herbal tea

Snack

150 g (5 oz) low-fat fruity fromage frais

Lunch

 RECIPE
Tomato bruschetta
Piece of fruit

Snack

2 tablespoons extra-light cream cheese mixed with 1 teaspoon pesto and 4 chopped olives, and served with 3 breadsticks

Evening Meal

RECIPE
Baked sweet potato with avocado and chilli topping

Strawberries and quark

250 g (8 oz) fresh strawberries, chopped
1 tablespoon balsamic vinegar
1 teaspoon caster sugar
2 ginger biscuits, roughly crushed
1 tablespoon quark

Place the strawberries in a small bowl, then drizzle the balsamic vinegar over the top. Dust with the caster sugar, scatter the ginger biscuits over the top and serve with a dollop of quark.

tomato bruschetta

Serves 1   Kcal 269   Protein 16 g   Carbs 30   Fat 10 g

12 cherry tomatoes
50 g (2 oz) mozzarella
  cheese

3 thick slices of ciabatta
olive oil, for brushing
a few basil leaves

1   Chop the cherry tomatoes into small pieces and thinly slice the mozzarella. Set aside.

2   Brush the ciabatta with a little oil, then arrange the sliced mozzarella and chopped cherry tomatoes on the toast. Tear the basil leaves into small pieces and scatter over the bruschetta.

3   Toast under a preheated hot grill until the cheese has melted slightly and serve immediately.

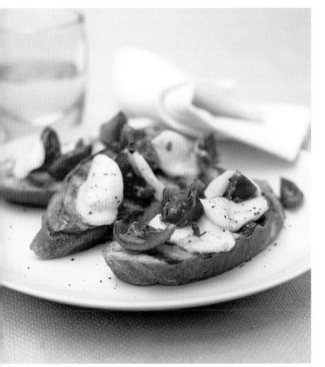

baked sweet potato with avocado and chilli topping

Serves 1   Kcal 371   Protein 8 g   Carbs 47 g   Fat 17 g

1 sweet potato, about
  200 g (7 oz)
1/2 small avocado, chopped
1/2 red chilli, finely
  chopped

1/2 red onion, chopped
2 tomatoes, chopped
15 g (1/2 oz) Emmental
  cheese, grated

1   Bake the sweet potato in a preheated oven at 200°C/400°F/Gas Mark 6 for 45–60 minutes or until tender. Halve lengthways when cool enough to touch.

2   In a bowl, mix together the avocado, red chilli, red onion, tomatoes and Emmental and spoon over the potato halves.

3   Place under a preheated hot grill for 2–3 minutes until the cheese is golden and bubbling. Serve with a green salad.

Chilli lovers take note
Not only do chillies provide body-protecting antioxidants, they also relieve nasal congestion, temporarily boost metabolism and trigger 'feel-good' chemicals in the brain called endorphins – which helps explain some people's undying devotion to them.

questions and answers

Q1 Why do I crave chocolate so much?

Chocolate is the most craved of all foods, and tastes fantastic. Cravings tend to happen if you feel you must restrict highly desirable foods such as chocolate – the 'naughty but nice' factor. Then there is its melt-in-the-mouth more-ishness and the finding that this pleasure stimulates the release of 'feel-good' brain chemicals 'endorphins'. You then start to link eating chocolate with feeling better and automatically turn to it or crave it for comfort.

Q2 If I stay up until 5 am, why do I start to feel more awake?

Known as your 'second wind', this happens because at that time of the day your body clock naturally starts to gear your body to move from sleep to being awake and alert (body temperature and adrenaline levels slowly start to rise) – even though you haven't actually slept!

Q3 Is the body clock way of eating suitable for the whole family?

Yes it is. But rather than follow the meal plans exactly, use them as a basis for family meals (increase quantities according to the number of people) and include more energy-giving carbohydrates, dairy foods and snacks for growing children and those with big, active appetites. After all, eating regular balanced meals and snacks, with plenty of fruit and vegetables, is healthy for everyone. You can adapt family favourites too (see pages 54–55).

Q4 Can I still eat out on the body clock diet?

Yes you can. The body clock approach isn't just a 'diet', but a guide to healthier eating for life. If you eat out a lot (this includes buying snacks and ready meals from sandwich bars and cafés), then you will need to make some changes. Food eaten away from home is generally higher in fat and calories and easy to view as a treat – so you feel it's fine to eat loads. If it is a very occasional treat, then enjoy. But successful slimmers limit fast food and cook at home more often. If you eat out at least once a week, follow these tips:

1 Skip high-fat pastry, deep-fried, battered or 'crispy' foods, fatty meats, mayonnaise, rich dressings, butter, cream or cheese sauces. Opt for 'healthy choice' sandwiches

2 Request how you would like a dish cooked or served. Ask for any sauces or salad dressing 'on the side', so you can add to taste – or ask for fat-free dressings

3 Order plenty of vegetables or salad – without added butter or oily dressings

4 Don't feel you have to finish everything on your plate. Food is more of a waste if you eat it when you don't want it

5 Avoid restaurants serving 'all-you-can-eat' buffets. Go for places that you know offer healthier choices. An increasing number provide nutritional information too

Q5 What if I am on a special diet?

If you need a special diet for medical reasons, then you must follow the advice of your doctor and dietitian. But since the body clock approach is based on healthy eating guidelines, it should suit most people who have conditions such as diabetes, high blood pressure or high cholesterol. But check with your doctor first before starting this or any other weight-loss approach. If you have a food intolerance, then you could still use the body clock principles, but substitute suitable foods as required.

Q6 How can I eat healthily when I work late?

If you work long hours, you may find that you are so hungry by the end of the day it's difficult to have the discipline to eat healthily. The best thing to do is to remember to have another snack later at work. Keep good choices in your work kitchen, desk drawer or bag, whichever

suits best. Make it part of your evening meal, say vegetable soup, a bean or fruit salad or fruit plus yogurt or a pot of rice pudding – so you just skip that part when you finally get home.

Q7 I feel stressed and often get up in the night and eat. This helps me relax and sleep, but is making me fat. What can I do about it?

You may have a problem with night eating. This is when people tend to skip breakfast, have little during the day and eat most of their food later on, and into the night, especially if they have trouble sleeping. Eating seems to help with stress and sleep, and studies suggest that people with 'night-eating syndrome' have an upset in their circadian rhythm of food intake along with their appetite, sleep and metabolism-regulating hormones. A first step is to stabilize your eating by having regular meals, starting with breakfast – body clock style. Initially, aim simply to keep your weight stable rather than lose any – you can move on to that when you feel more in control. Look for ways to help you relax, especially before bed (see page 46), to help you sleep regularly too. Physical activity during the day also helps (see page 32). If there is no improvement, then do see your doctor to discuss treatment options.

Q8 I think I may have SAD, as I feel flat in the winter and comfort eat. What can I do?

Most of us feel better when the sun is shining; grey gloom can sap spirits, making us slow down – and eat more. For some, this can go to the extremes of seasonal affective disorder (SAD), which may affect up to 3 per cent of the population during winter months (SAD is rare in countries nearer the equator) and is three times more common amongst women. Then there is a milder version, referred to as 'subsyndromal SAD' or 'winter blues'.

Symptoms of SAD include low mood, sleep problems, carbohydrate or 'comfort food' cravings, lethargy, weight gain and anxiety. It is usually helped with light therapy, a healthy diet based on regular meals, regular exercise and counselling. More research is needed, but SAD seems to be caused in susceptible people by not getting enough light in the winter to keep up levels of chemical messengers such as the mood and sleep regulators serotonin and melatonin. It could also be a sign of a delayed body clock. So do talk to your doctor if your mood is low, or you think you may have SAD. The lifestyle basics of the body clock approach can also help SAD, and the more common 'winter blues'.

Q9 Is food eaten late at night more fattening?

Studies have shown that a large meal eaten late at night does not make the body store more fat than smaller meals over the day – it is the total amount you eat in a 24-hour period that is important. However, people who skip meals during the day, get starving hungry, then eat loads late in the evening are more likely to be overweight than regular meal eaters because they are out of sync with their natural appetite regulators. Frequently eating most of your calories late in the night may also make the body more resistant to blood sugar-regulating insulin. This can make it harder for people to manage their weight.

Q10 I haven't lost any more weight for three weeks. How can I get going again?

Weight plateaus are common – the trick is to stay realistic and keep up the positive 'self-talk' (see page 43). It could be that you have come close to your natural 'settling' weight, so check that you don't have an unachievable weight goal or are expecting to lose weight too quickly. If not, then keep your food and thoughts diary (see page 40). It is very easy to slip back into old habits or eat that bit more. Could you be more active too? That really makes a difference. Keep in regular contact with your supporters; you truly need them now. If you have addressed all these things, and you have already lost at least 10 kg (1½ stones), then you may need to adjust your diet a bit (see page 45), since there is less of you burning energy day to day. Remember that staying positive and believing in yourself is the key.

Q11 I have a slow metabolism and can't lose weight. Will the body clock diet help me?

Research is now clear that overweight people actually have a higher metabolic rate than lighter people. This is because heavier bodies use more energy or calories to function and move around. What can make it harder for some people though are genetic differences in things like levels of appetite-regulating hormones, being spontaneously active, even food preferences. The body clock approach will help you to address all of these things – so, as for any approach based on healthy living, it will help in many ways.

Q12 Do I need to take vitamin supplements?

The body clock diet meal plans are very well balanced. But whenever you change what you eat, taking a one-a-day vitamin and mineral supplement is a good back-up, especially for women.

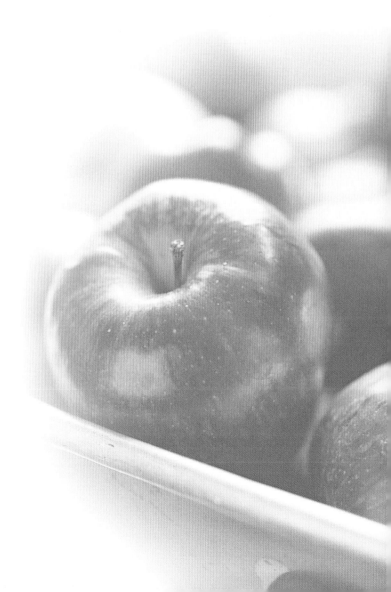

index

acknowledgements

Author's acknowledgements
With special thanks to:
Dr Clare Grace, Research Dietitian, Royal London Hospital
Dax Moy, Corrective and Performance Exercise Specialist, London
Gaynor Bussell, Women's Health Dietitian and adviser for the National Association for Premenstrual Syndrome (NAPS), UK
Linda Bird, health and lifestyle writer, and author of the *Weekend Home Spa*

Publisher's acknowledgements
Recipes Louise Blair
Executive Editor Jane McIntosh
Editor Alice Tyler
Executive Art Editor Leigh Jones
Designer Miranda Harvey
Photography Gareth Sambidge
Stylist Liz Hippisley
Home Economy Lucy McKelvie and Emma McIntosh
Picture Researcher Jennifer Veall
Production Controller Martin Croshaw

Picture acknowledgements
Getty Images/31, 32, 44, 47 /Antony Nagelmann 28/Charles Thatcher 63/Ken Fisher 48/Laurence Monneret 4–5/Steve Smith 17
Octopus Publishing Group Limited
/Craig Robertson 23 /William Lingwood 27/David Munns 19/Peter Pugh-Cook 35, 43, 52 /Russell Sadur 1, 7, 41 /Ian Wallace 15, 22, 25, 81, 109